MW01253819

Vital Health Nutrition

How to Become Healthy
in a Crazy Western Society

David S. Lee

Hon. Bsc., Bed., B.R.E., N.H.C., CPTN.
Certified Naturotherapist, Shiatsu Therapist, Iridologist,
Bio-Nutritionist and Western/Chinese Herbalist

VITAL HEALTH NUTRITION:
HOW TO BECOME HEALTHY IN A CRAZY WESTERN SOCIETY,
by David S. Lee.

ISBN 978-0-9949222-0-5

In memory
of my dear mentor and friend
Julian Beecroft

Contents

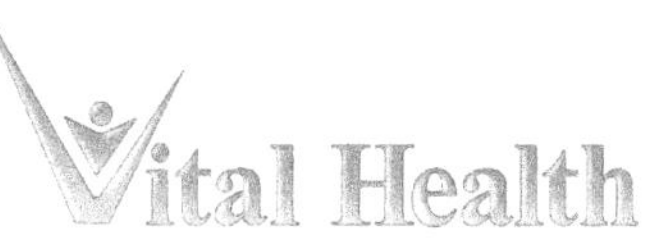
Vital Health

Acknowledgments

I would like to deeply thank the following people:

Linda Tanguay, for her tireless and consistent help with formatting and word processing functions;

My teachers at the International Academy of Natural Health Science, especially John Freeman, Cecile Savereux and Dr. Dorothy Marshall, for their encouraging and insightful teachings; Dr. George Grant for guiding me through his vast knowledge of medical science and nutritional bio-chemistry; Diane Samulski for always introducing new and exciting health supplements, foods and empowering activities; Todd Norton for his friendship, encouragement and input on health issues and bio-nutritional facts; Tonie and Luis Rivas for being there as friends and supporting me in various health endeavours;

David Kujawa for all his technical advice on how to take good pictures; Alex Barker for his help with book design; Rosemary Knes for her professional editing help;

My dear Clelia DeMarinas, who was like a mother to me and always had a listening ear and an open heart to hear the things I had to say;

My GIN friends, Symeon Rogers and Muhammad Salad for their help and support;

Bill Garbarino for his friendship, steadfast guidance, and wise business counsel over the years through the various circumstances and development of Vital Health;

My dear sister, Ella, who always believed in me, supported my vision and encouraged me during those challenging times in my life when I had to clarify my dreams;

My late mentor and friend, James Stockton, who was like an earthly Christ figure in my life, who impacted my thoughts and life with not just his wise words but his everyday example of loving people and giving;

And my late mentor and father figure, Julian, who exposed me to healthy foods, and for birthing many of the health and fitness ideas which I developed further into the Vital Health System.

Preface

I wrote this book to help people understand that weight loss is not about jumping on the latest fad or following a quick, product-driven diet or an extreme calorie reduced regiment. It's not about counting calories with point systems or packaged, low-calorie frozen food that you have to purchase along with a program.

It's about transforming your perception of yourself. It's about knowing you are worthwhile and valuable enough to spend energy and time to cook yourself wonderful, healthy meals, and to exercise, stretch and move your body so that it becomes strong, supple, lean, agile and fit. It's about looking after your "temple" (your body) where you experience your life day to day. Your body is the centre of your world. If it does not work well or feel well, then your experience of everyday life is greatly limited.

It's about a lifestyle change that starts with a mental shift in your thinking. It's about making a clear life plan and life-changing decisions that you slowly acquire in the process of transforming your habits and ways of thinking about food, drink and activities. It's about learning that whole, natural foods are out there for you to enjoy and to cook and prepare. It's about learning easy recipes and meals that fuel your body with amazing energy. It's about experiencing mental sharpness and clarity of thought and a sense of well being that will give you a secure sense of peace; one that says you are on the right path.

My Holistic Health Philosophy

BEING HEALTHY MAKES US FEEL GOOD

Eckhart Tolle talks about living in the "Now" mentally as we live our lives day to day.[1] If you think about how in nature our days and nights pass by, it's like each day is a chapter of a story in a comic book. We start our day as the sun rises from the east. We get up and carry out our activities based on the thoughts we think, emotions we feel and the beliefs we have about ourselves and the beliefs of what we think is right or wrong, consciously or subconsciously. Every day we decide what we believe is possible, then we commit to it consciously, or at times subconsciously, and follow through with action to succeed. We do this as human beings because it makes us feel good. There is nothing more exciting than when we achieve our dreams or are in the process of getting there!

The weather, the temperature, and all of nature and creation around us are seen as changes in colours, shapes, and sounds. We are breathing human organisms in the midst of it all, taking in the entire stimulus coming at us minute by minute. If we pay attention to each detail of all that is happening, it can be overwhelming. All the mysterious manifestations of the world, good and bad, displays itself each chapter of each day. What's even more amazing is we are given the ability to create our day with our intentions of what we want to feel and experience moment to moment. We make choices, either consciously or subconsciously, of what we want, how we want it, where we want it, etc. We usually gravitate towards things, people, events and situations that make us feel good and usually move away from things, events, people and situations that make us feel bad.[2]

This is one of the reasons why being healthy and fit plays such an important role in making us feel good about ourselves, about our life in general, and about approaching others. When we nourish our bodies properly, we take on the positive mood effects of hormones such as Insulin, Serotonin and Dopamine. We feel better about ourselves. You cannot get away from the way your body works and feels to how you experience your life!

DYSFUNCTION IN OUR SOCIETY

I'm sure you have wondered at some point how all the processed foods out there affect our health, especially our digestion. A significant portion of our foods are GMO (Genetically Modified Organisms), irradiated and processed with all kinds of food flavorings, colour and preservatives. As a society, we are not educated on how this affects our bodies on the inside, nor do people seem to care enough to learn about the foods they eat. As long as it tastes good and the commercials confirm it is "wholesome and good for you", most people unconsciously buy into it and find themselves in the fast-food lineup. People will spend more energy and research into buying a new car – a depreciating asset that will eventually rust out and will have to be replaced – and buying what's on sale with little resistance than on the food they put into their mouths. However, with our bodies, we don't get a second chance. You can't trade it in for a better model. I look at many older people sitting in doctors' offices, getting medications, hanging on to every word doctors say, but never looking at the option of taking control of their own health before it is too late. Unfortunately, we as a society that has been programmed by the media, food industries and much of the medical system to count calories, go to the gym and take the medications prescribed for ailing digestion, stomach, and joints. Pardon me for my directness, but when are we going to WAKE UP! When are we going to realize there is something wrong here! Because of this state of affairs, I have written this Vital Health Nutrition book as a way of educating and increasing your awareness so you can take more control of your health.

Vital Health Nutrition consists of a five-step program of cleanses that resets your hormonal levels, infuses your body with needed enzymes that breakdown food and introduces hundreds of micronutrients from the raw whole foods to the cells of your body. Also, I will give you a list of things to do on a regular basis to not only lose weight, but to keep you at optimal health. The guidelines of this book will show you how to get rid of the toxins and possibly some parasites in your body, nourish yourself properly with well combined foods in a meal plan, lose the excess fat and keep your muscle by eating a hormonally balanced meal plan, always combined with whole, raw foods full of micronutrients. I will also show you how to decrease your stress levels by practicing a short meditation exercise of deep breathing that will help renew your mind and allow you to let go of that tendency to live in the future or the past. It will cause you to focus more on the present moments of your life, so that daily life becomes more enjoyable, fulfilling, and peaceful.

HEALTH AND NUTRITION IS THE KEY

You don't need to look too far to see the physical state most people are in, and realize people don't seem to be getting healthier, even though we have health clubs everywhere with state-of-the-art equipment. The statistics from the past 20 years show people across North America are getting fatter and weaker, with a significant percentage struggling with heart diseases, cancer and diabetes. The refined, un-organic flour foods people consume in the form of muffins, bagels, breads, etc. are affecting our bodies in negative ways; not to mention how this has contributed to the obesity challenge in North America.[3]

As I trained clients over the years, I became increasingly concerned and frustrated because even though they progressed in strength and lost some weight, their overall health was poor. There was a lack of attention to nutrition, sleep patterns, stress levels and negative lifestyle habits. The reason why so many people are over-stressed is because they are not looking after one of the most important thing they possess: their body.

I think Bill Phillips said it best in his book Body for Life, "*When I see women and men out of shape physically, unhealthy, I see lives not fully lived, I see lost potential, I see people who need someone to help them realize they can look and feel better. You can't escape this reality; your body is the epicentre of your universe!*"[4]

With the onslaught of the technological age, people have become weaker and fatter because of less physical activity, therefore less muscle tissue, hence less strength. The new term that is used is Sarcopenia which is the loss of lean body mass (muscle) to the point your body composition changes from less muscle and higher fat in percentage terms even though you may weigh the same. If this continues as you age, the onset of osteoporosis is one of the results. As people reach their elderly years, another result is they become weak because of the lack of muscle tissue and they are unable to perform day-to-day functional tasks on their own anymore. Hence, they unnecessarily end up in assisted living residences.[5]

As I worked with my clients over the years, a significant number of them could not progress past a certain point in the training programs. Their unhealthy lifestyles outside the gym, eating habits and their chronic health issues slowed down their progress significantly and in some cases brought them back to the same place they were when we started. In a number of cases, they could not continue because their health issues increased and they were unable to function well enough to participate in the program. Unfortunately, I had clients that made changes in my programs, but did not go all the way in eliminating habits that can actually shorten your life, such as smoking. I attended the funeral of one client who was not even 50 years old. Even though she was eating better and exercising, the smoking caught up with her. When she defaulted to some of the not-so-healthy lifestyle patterns, her immune system dropped and cancer occurred. Her doctors said she had had the cancer for a period of time before it manifested, but it was dormant because her immune system had kept it under control.

INFLAMMATION AND HORMONAL IMBALANCE

Poor diet plays havoc on energy levels and leads to a host of health issues, which are directly or indirectly caused by an imbalance of chemical messengers called hormones that are produced by the various endocrine glands of the body. The hormones of the endocrine system respond to the internal changes of our body, taking minutes, hours or even days before you see their effects.[6] The pituitary gland referred to as the "master gland" produces its hormones which act on the thyroid glands, ovaries, testes and adrenal glands to regulate growth, reproduction, nutrient absorption and metabolism. Each of these secretes their own hormones. For instance, ovaries and testes secrete the sex hormones estrogen, progesterone and testosterone. The adrenal glands secrete cortisol and the anti-stress hormone DHEA. The thyroid releases thyroid hormones that manage metabolism. Hormones also affect body shape and appearance, skin, and hair. They also control appetite and affect metabolism which greatly plays an important role in fat loss.

For the purposes of this book, I want to look at how poor nutrition and lifestyle can bring about the negative effects of inflammation in the body, hormonal imbalance in Insulin, cortisol, estrogen, thyroid and high stress which bring on the health symptoms so common today in our society.

When there is inflammation anywhere in the body, digestive issues, stress and poor sleeping habits, the various hormones that play a role in that organ or system either increase or decrease in their levels which then leads to a host of other symptoms. Inflammation of the digestive system is one of the main health challenges that Vital Health Nutrition looks after. The reason for this focus is about 60% of your immune system is affected by your digestive tract! Such things as food allergies, not enough good bacteria, low levels of enzymes and acids, yeast growth like Candida, high parasite levels and stress affect your digestion which, in turn, affects the whole immune system. When the immune system is overtaxed from chronic infections, emotional stress, and exposure to harmful toxins, inflammation can occur in the body. Poor eating habits such as consuming too many carbohydrates made with refined sugar will cause inflammation.

 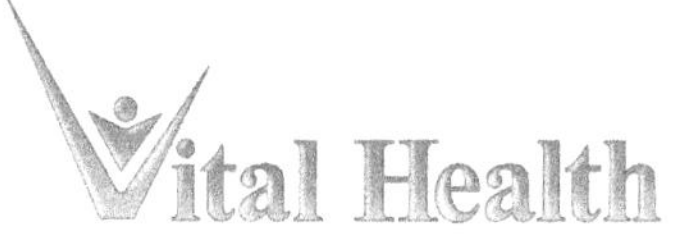

One of the main health issues many people experience is an excess of insulin occurring from too much of these kinds of carbohydrates. When insulin is released in the blood stream, it is directed in three ways:

1. It is immediately used as fuel; a large portion by the brain and kidneys;
2. It is stored as glycogen in the liver or muscles for later use as an energy source;
3. It stores any excess sugar as fat if the glycogen stores are already full and not being immediately used, as in going for an hour run after having dessert.

This is why you need to be careful on the amount of high-sugar and high carbohydrate foods, especially if you do not want to gain excess fat or if you are trying to lose weight.

Another hormone which plays a huge role in our body is cortisol which is secreted by the adrenal glands located on top of your kidneys. Under persistent chronic stress whether physical, mental, emotional or environmental, real or imagined, the body will release high amounts of cortisol. If you have chronic health issues like Irritable Bowel Syndrome (IBS) causing stress on your digestion, your cortisol levels will be high. Unfortunately, excess cortisol will use up muscle tissue for fuel, whereas adrenalin will use fat stores for energy. Therefore, long periods of stress can lead to muscle wasting and high blood sugar which leads to fat gain, fatigue, and decrease in strength. However, cortisol like adrenalin also has a positive role in the body. It helps us adapt to stressful situations like maintaining our blood pressure, body temperature, and controls inflammation.

Estrogen is produced primarily in the ovaries of women before menopause and by the adrenal glands and fat cells after menopause. It plays a crucial role in the menstruation cycle by building up the tissue and blood in the uterus. It is considered mainly a female hormone, but it is important for men as well. However, when men gain too much fat, their fat cells start to convert testosterone to estrogen. Too much alcohol and a high-fat diet also causes excess levels of estrogen in both men and women. When this happens, a condition called estrogen dominance occurs which causes toxic fat gain, water retention, bloating, and a host of other health issues.

I have been talking about the havoc negative stress can have on our bodies. But there is also a positive level of stress we all need, like exercise, running or playing a sport. However, if that stress is prolonged to an excess, the body will be unable to handle it. You can see this in professional and recreational athletes who over-train. When you push your body to fatigue three to four times a week for an hour and a half at the gym on top of a full-time job, it is easy for the stress on the body to go past the point of being positive to become a negative stressor. Hence, the immune system drops and you end up catching whatever "bug" is in the air and a cold or flu usually occurs. This is where it is really important to listen to your body's signals and how you feel to make sure you are getting enough down time. Be aware of how stiff you are, how tight or loose your muscles feel. When you are fully recuperated, your muscles feel tight and your veins pop out very easily and you feel stronger in your contractions, not to mention your motivation to want to train is higher. When I mean down time, I mean staying home in a quiet atmosphere, soft music playing and doing a lot of lying down on the couch with feet up, reading a book, watching movies, etc. Personally, when I am training a lot – usually three to four times a week with jogging/running seven to 10 Km three times a week in addition to the gym work and doing my core and floor work five to six days a week – I make sure I have regular rest times to recuperate. I literally spend up to three or four hours of just lying down in a very relaxed state every evening to recuperate. Without this time, you will start getting sick and end up with injuries because the body is not recuperating and the muscles need to regain their glycogen levels completely.

MENTAL AND SPIRITUAL PRACTICES

Some of the things I find helpful in lowering stress levels is to do short 10-minute meditations every few days, set goals using a Life Plan, practice three- to five-minute visualizations every morning of what you want in your life and what you want to achieve. These practices will increase your belief that you can be, do, or have anything you want. The exercise sheets at the beginning of this book, like The Life Plan, Healthy Thinking for Life, Life Style Habits & Behaviour and Positive Statements and Empowering Questions, will help you identify your

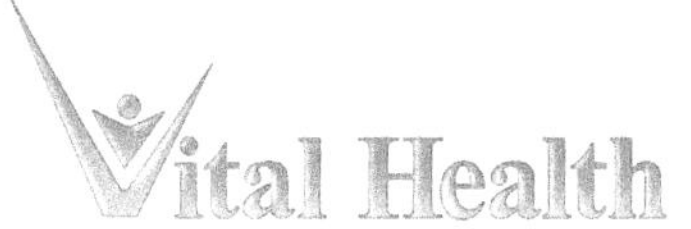

values which fuel your goals, re-evaluate your habits, prioritize and increase your belief that you can be the healthiest you've ever been and be in the best shape of your life!

You can do meditations for 10 to 15 minutes in your room, or on your bed in the morning as soon as you get up. This is a good time because your brain is still in an alpha phase which is a meditative state. Also, you can repeat positive affirmations in this state so it eventually ends up in the subconscious beliefs of your heart, which is the centre from where you operate your life. I personally have done this for a few years. As I repeated healing phrases and sentences to replace the negative ones I had in my heart, it allowed me to get rid of negative beliefs I had about myself and others. I learned much of this from an amazing teacher, Dr. James B. Richards, from his Heart Physics program which he talks about in his book, Wired for Success, Programmed for Failure.[7]

Setting your goals in writing makes a huge difference in achieving them because you took the time to mentally process your goals. I have developed a mental exercise template called a Life Plan which I personally used to reach my personal and business goals. It has brought much harmony and confidence. You will go through all the details on how to do this in the next section.

I would like to explain more in detail how to do the visualizations. The technique I use is a short visualization with eyes closed for three to five minutes at the beginning of each day. I use the main goal I am working towards in my life at that time. It's good to visualize in colour and try to even imagine the sounds and smells that are associated with what you are visualizing. The more real you make it, the stronger it will pull in that thing you want from the Universe. This practice works with the concept of "The Law of Attraction", which I'm sure you've heard of as it is one of the main topics introduced in the movie "The Secret". I strongly recommend you read "Ask and It is Given", written by Esther and Jerry Hicks if you want to know how the Law of Attraction works energetically. As I mentioned earlier, I believe we create the reality of our lives by what we think about, focus on, talk about, and send intentions to. Think about loving people, about positive things, and you will attract into your life wonderful positive people, events and situations. Think negatively – you're bitter about someone, you have a lot of resentment, fear and hatred – and you will attract similar people, situations and events. I hope you choose to always think, visualize and say positive things.

BACK TO NUTRITIONAL TOPICS

I am convinced, after research, attending seminars, consulting with doctors and health specialists, that what people consume as food and drink is a huge factor that contributes to strength, recovery, healing, stamina, mental sharpness and energy. I have seen that when my clients over the past 16 years ate more enzyme rich foods, foods rich in omega-3, higher in fibre, higher in minerals, vitamins, micronutrients and organic foods where possible, their bodies began to restore to a healthier balance, eliminating or decreasing the symptoms they were suffering from.[8] They became more positive-oriented people with a more positive outlook on life. Therefore, I have developed this Vital Health System of nutrition for people to use as a guide to how they should eat 80 to 90 percent of the time to keep the body strong, with a high immune system that will keep them disease free and allow them to age gracefully with higher energy, vitality, and stamina.

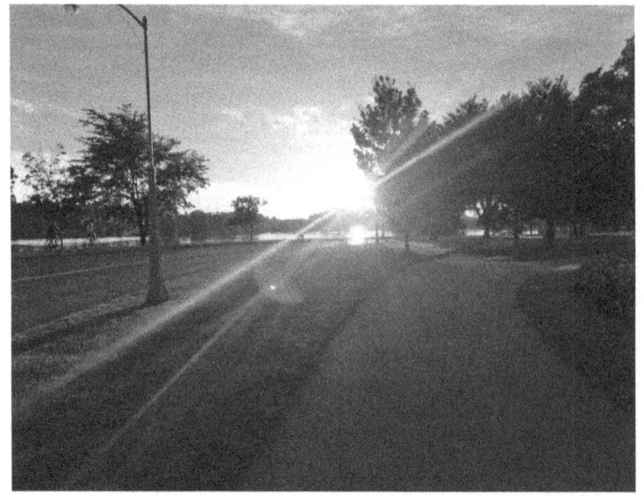

Life Plan

I have come to the conclusion that for people to make the mental shift necessary to commit to a lifestyle change of exercise and healthy eating – that is spending time in the gym or at home, going for walks and jogs and taking time to prepare healthier meals – they need to really look at the reasons why they are doing this and clarify the value it gives them. Without a true heartfelt conviction of knowing you are doing the right thing for yourself, it will be easy for you to quit or get distracted. Therefore, I have provided copies of mental exercise sheets so you can define a plan of how you want to live your life from this moment on. This is called a Life Plan. The plan can be an extension of how you feel and think. Just the act of writing your thoughts, goals and dreams down on paper will stimulate around 10,000 neural pathways in your brain.[9] Look around you at people as they talk. Their whole body changes in movement, gesture of hands, fingers, etc. They physically change as the mood or the tone of their words change. You will also have a higher recollection of your thoughts by writing it down than typing it on a computer.[10] This is why I suggest you print off the Life Plan section of this book and fill in the various sections of the plan by hand writing. Then if you wish, you can type it all into your computer for future editing. As you change your habits and become more of a health conscious individual, you will need to do some extra mental work on the other aspects of your life.

In my 16 years of experience in the personal training and nutrition consulting business, one of the main reasons many clients could not continue on the fitness/

nutrition program was because other areas of their life would end up unravelling and they could not focus on their goal of becoming healthier and fitter. Either it was financial challenges, relationship issues or work demands on their time. It's almost as if most people sabotage their success when it comes to getting healthier and fit. There is a lack of focus in their life on what it is that they want and what priorities they really have. I need to help you reprogram yourself so you don't end up falling off track half way along your journey in this decision. There is a statement I learned and that is "success is a decision away". We need to get you thinking of yourself as being successful in this new life style change. The thinking is what got you into an unhealthy lifestyle to begin with, so now we need to reverse that program in your mind and have you think in terms of embracing all the changes that will be happening in your experience as you start to eat well, look better, cook healthier and exercise more. What many people don't know is that there is a universal law that works similarily to this statement, made by a famous success coach, Harvey Ecker, "How we do anything is how we do everything".[11] What this is saying is how you carry out your commitment in one aspect of your life will have a spillover effect on other aspects of your life. A lot of people do things with "a poke it with a stick method" instead of being fully onboard and commit to what they have decided no matter what!

LIFE PLAN AS A TOOL

The Life Plan is a great tool in making a fairly detailed plan on what kind of life you want to live day to day, in all areas of your life; with a healthy focus on proper eating and exercise to look after your God-given body. This also allows you to see that you create your life as you go, by the way you think, and the choices you make every minute. The universe responds to your demands and intentions, be they negative or positive. That is why you want to be careful what kinds of thoughts you dwell on, what kind of words you say about yourself and others. If you think positive, encouraging thoughts about yourself and others. That is what you are going to attract. Both Thomas Edison and Albert Einstein said, "Our brain is a transmitter and receiver of frequencies!" When you think a thought you are sending a frequency. Top scientists have proven that the law of attraction is a real force at work in all of our lives.[12] We are all energy! Based on the latest quantum physics research, this is now an accepted fact among most of the scientific community.[13]

WHAT DO YOU VALUE?

In the first section, I'd like you to come up with at least six values that you live your life by. For example, what is your value regarding money? Do you value that you should always live within your means and save money for the future? What is your value in terms of friendships? Do you believe in having and maintaining one or two close friendships? In regards to the environment you want to live in, do you value living closer to nature or are you happier in a bustling city where there is lots of excitement and adventure? What kind of character traits do you value in people that you want to associate with? Do you value a person who is humble, reliable, always does what they say they will do? I think this should give you a pretty good idea of what values you can come up with.

HOW DO YOU WANT YOUR LIFE TO LOOK LIKE?

This section is going to cover what you want your life to look like in its various components. Here, you will start to make decisions to create the life you want to live, based on the values you have defined and concluded were the most important to you.

FINANCIALLY

Let's start with your financial situation. How do you want that to be, based on the values you have defined? For example, you want to always have enough money to travel and enjoy, experience some of your dreams every three months or so; or you may want to just be able to treat yourself every month at a nice restaurant without worrying about the bill, or to buy those expensive sunglasses or buy front seat tickets to see your favourite band, like U2. Tickets for you and your partner or a friend to a U2 concert can be a hefty sum, from what I have heard; worth saving for.

So here I want to show you how to create a budget plan where you set a percentage of money aside towards that expenditure every time you get paid and the rest stays in your chequing account to look after your bills. This is where I change gears as I show you how to budget your weekly pay and open up seven to eight accounts. I personally have followed this budgeting system and it has been very liberating and helped me enjoy my money more and also save. If you have a business, you will need to open up eight accounts. If you have a job, then you will only need to open seven accounts because your employer deducts the tax from your pay. The banks usually allow you to have a chequing and savings account. Then you can set up another six savings-type accounts which you can access online under "other" account.

I personally learned this from a motivational success course created by T. Harvey Eker. Here is an example of the budget for a person in business living off their gross income:

17% aside for taxes

6% for play fund (you spend this every month or so, on a gift or treat for yourself)

3% for contingencies (emergency expenses that may arise, i.e. flat tire, car repair)

6% for holidays (spend every three months or so for a weekend trip, hotel, or cruise, etc.)

3% education fund (books, audios, events, courses, seminars that help you grow as a person)

3% giving fund to a charity of your choice, or to a cause

10% for short-term savings (to buy a new car, new wardrobe, new boat)

10% for long-term savings (for a house, cottage, retirement, etc.)

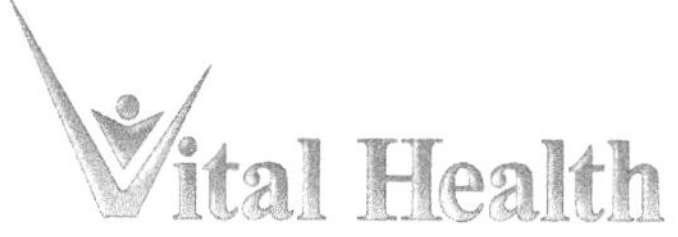

This budget system, if you apply it, will start to stabilize your financial life so that you can pursue and carry out the fitness and health program you are learning in this book. So you can afford the gym membership you may buy in the process, or even buy some fitness equipment to set up your own exercise space in your home. One of the main ideas I learned from this system of budgeting was that we need to enjoy our money regularly, by spending a portion of it on whatever makes you feel good! Actually, what you are doing is feeling "rich" for a few hours or a day because you are just going to spend the whole amount in that "play fund" account and not feel guilty about it. It sends out a message to the universe that you are willing to receive abundance into your life, so the universe will bring more situations, people and things to make you richer! Another example of the Law of Attraction at work!

SOCIALLY

Now let us look at your social life. Do you want friends who are going to be supportive of your healthy lifestyle change, be a positive influence in your life and not be a negative drain? I'm not crazy about waking you up to this fact but science has proven that we end up with the average income of our five best friends.[14] What this means is you are greatly influenced by the people you hang out with in your life. Hence, if you are not becoming successful in your life or it seems like you are stuck and not moving forward in your life, you may need to look at the type of friends you are hanging out with! Write out a plan of action of how many times a month you want to get together with some new positive, successful people, or do things with a new acquaintance who is successful in some way and has a lot of the positive qualities you want. As time goes, it will rub off on you! Take action and call them within 48 hours and do something because when we don't take action on a decision within 48 hours, we start to regress.[15] There is also an association I am a part of called the Global Information Network (GIN) which is mainly a society of like-minded people who want to grow mentally, spiritually and in their character so they become successful in all aspects of their life. Their website is at: globalinformationnetwork.com.

EMOTIONALLY

The next section is a very important one since it's dealing with your state of emotions. How do you want to feel everyday – emotionally – most of the time? I realize there will be days when you may feel bad about something; maybe you are laid off, or someone in your family dies, etc. Life happens around you. How do you want to respond to those things that occur in the external world? What kind of emotions do you want to feel every day? Do you want to feel powerful, fit, full of energy, and ready to take on world? You have to live within your internal world, and that is where the universe will respond in your life. Define the specific emotions you want to feel; like joyful, exhilarated, motivated, anticipating something good is going to come your way, feeling sexy, beautiful, tranquil, at peace, enlightened, in a constant state of enlightenment about life around you, feeling like a winner, feeling valued, respected, etc. You want to think about those emotions you feel on your most happy days. Think about the days you've had in the past that were the most memorable days, where you felt you were on top of the world, living life to the fullest and doing the things that made you feel really good. Start by identifying those emotions you felt during those times and write them in as the emotions you want to feel most of the time in your life plan.

PHYSICALLY

This section is where I think a lot of people have challenges because it's the one thing that everyone says they want, but their focus, commitment and ability to persevere of staying fit usually goes to the sidelines, because as other distractions

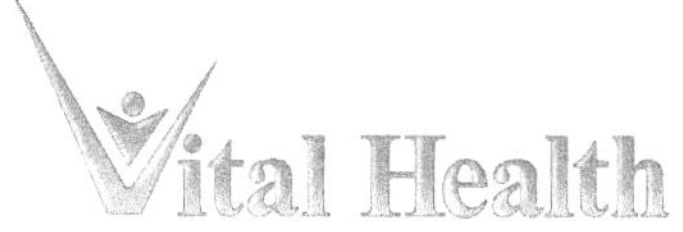

come in during the course of a day, most people push it aside. However, staying healthy and fit is probably one of the main factors in being able to experience life and enjoying it at an optimal level. If you are carrying an excess 20 pounds, you tend to avoid mirrors, don't feel as beautiful, wear clothes to hide and your energy levels are not as good. Think about what it would feel like if you strapped an extra 20 pound plate of weight to your body and walked around all day. Would you not start to feel worn out more from moving around with that extra burden coming down on all your joints, back, hips, etc.? I want you to define exactly how much weight you need to trim off your body to look and feel your best. I want you to write down a rough timeline of when you want to reach that ideal body shape and fitness level because if you don't most people will tend not to reach it. You have to make a commitment to yourself and stay focused on that goal as a priority every day as you are making all your other decisions in life. This is what makes life interesting. This makes you get up every day with more purpose and it builds a greater confidence in you to become better, do better and empower yourself every time you do your exercises and make that salad or healthier meal. You become stronger inside and out!

If you are already a seasoned bodybuilder, fitness person or athlete and you have fallen off the track a bit, and getting into shape is something you have been doing for a long time, then write in a goal of what body fat percentage you want to get back to or how much stronger you want to be on the bar squat or bench in a month, or maybe you want to be able to jog or run 10km in less than an hour.

AT WORK OR BUSINESS

Another aspect of your life you want to plan out and define is how you want to experience every day at work or at your business. Since many of us spend around seven to eight hours at a place of work or business five days a week, it would make sense that you define how you want your work life to be like. Do you want it to be peaceful at work, where you get along with all your associates, and your employer is kind, generous with their resources and holiday pay? Or if you are looking to go into another new job or field of work, what kind of work would be your dream job? What hours do you want to work; how long of a lunch break. Do you want to work for a company that has a great staffroom where you can warm up your food in the toaster oven, keep your lunch in the large fridge and sit at nicely decorated staff tables?

If it's a business of your own that you plan to have, then define what kind of an operation will make you the most fulfilled and happy. Do you want to always finish your business day by 4pm so you can do a workout at the gym and still have time to have dinner with your family? What kind of a secretary or staff would you like to hire? Do you want someone who is reliable, versatile and has great work ethics? I think you get the picture.

WORK ENVIRONMENT

This section is similar to the previous one, but I want you to define in detail what kind of environment you want to work in, as far as attitude, pace, expectations, kinds of people, etc. Do you want the attitudes of the staff to be complementary to yours or maybe you want them to have strengths in areas that you are weak in? For example, if you have great people skills, but are not great at technical computer software or hardware fixes, you may want to work with those who have better skills in that area. Do you want to be in a fast-paced work environment with lots of work to do or in a more laid-back kind of an environment like a library, where things are not as noisy or fast-paced as a bustling downtown coffee shop?

KIND OF HOME

What kind of things or experiences do you want to do at your home? Do you want it to be a place where it's like a safe haven, where you read, write letters, meditate

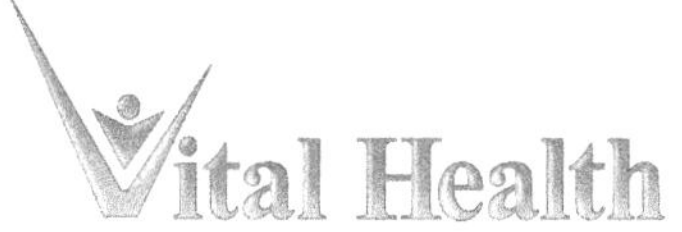

or do you want it to be set up for house guests on a regular basis, your family members coming to visit every month and staying over for the weekend? Everybody has different set-ups in their households. If you are part of a large, close family with lots of children, being able to have enough guest rooms to accommodate everybody will be important. Or if you are a single person who has a hectic job where you deal with lots of people all day, you may want your home to be more of a private place just for you.

KIND OF FITNESS FACILITY

If you are a real fitness person and don't have room for a home gym and you want to train at a club, what kind of a gym do you want to belong to? Do you want to be at a small cozy gym in a community centre where there are lots of family members with children, more laid-back, not as crowded? Or do you want to be at a big facility where there are hardcore people into training with lots of equipment to choose from? You may want to be part of a more Zen-like space where yoga and Pilates classes are held and where weight-training is not the focus.

SOCIAL ENVIRONMENT

At your regular social gatherings with friends and family or at social functions, such as a golf game or group card playing, how do you want to be a participant in that social experience? How do you want it to play out for you? Do you want to be with friends with whom you can share your cares and dreams and also offer a listening ear for them to share their dreams and goals? Define your ideal social experiences so that you walk away from them feeling great. We are basically made up of atoms which are basically energy. Therefore, keep away from people who are complainers, blamers and justifiers of why they are not successful at whatever they are making excuses for. Their negative energy will keep attracting other negative energy which means they will continue to perpetuate their own failure. If you continue to be with them too much, you will also be on the receiving end of the "crap".[16]

KIND OF SELF-NURTURE TIME

This section of the plan should cover what your special time alone is going to be like. Some people go for walks in the park, bike through the backwoods near their home or do laps in a salt-water pool for 30 minutes or so. You notice I emphasized "salt water" instead of the usual chlorine. Stay away from chlorinated water as much as possible because you can absorb it through your skin as you are swimming in it. It is too toxic for it to be a good thing especially to allow into your body when we are trying to get your body healthier! The amount of harm that has been reported in lab studies and cases are alarming such as skin rashes, kidney disorders, liver cancer, vision impairment, respiratory ailments, etc.[17]

HOW DO YOU WANT TO EXPERIENCE THESE THINGS?

In all the places you go every week to do your errands, like groceries, doctor's office, dental office, post office, gas station, coffee shop, health-food store, public transportation, etc., you have encounters with the people who work there. Since they are servicing you in some way, eventually, over time, you have to acknowledge them. How do you want to be with them in that exchange?

It can be easy for us to discount these experiences and people because they are not directly involved in our lives. But it is still a part of your life. We all are connected energetically in this universal web of matrix. Hence, we all affect each other in very subtle ways. These experiences become part of the fabric of our memory and we hold on to them and we will reminisce about them later in our life. Therefore, I make

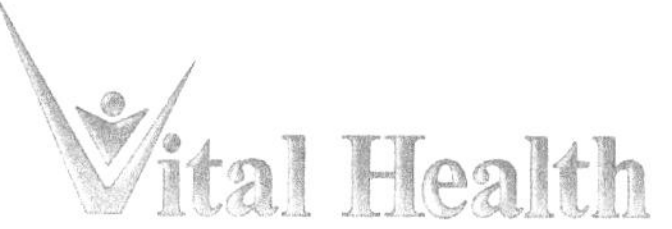

a point of being intentional as the creator of these experiences in how I respond and listen to those around me. If you really watch and take in the surroundings around you during these day-to-day – what may seem mundane – moments, they actually become magical. You may notice someone in the grocery store lineup, baby on their back; the baby smiles and you smile, maybe you shake a tiny hand. You take those few minutes to appreciate the gift of interacting with that baby's energy, a pure spirit, untainted by the world's distortions. It is part of how the universe, or God, shows us and reveals the love and harmony that exists in the world. You only need to take a moment to observe it with a grateful heart. You will find the reality of your day-to-day experience will change for the better in leaps and bounds! [18]

IF YOU HAD THE RESOURCES TO LIVE YOUR DREAM DAY

If you had all the money that you could ever want, how would you live each day or week starting from the moment you awaken to the minute you fall asleep? Describe it a step at a time as shown in the example.

PERSONAL GOALS

LEISURE GOALS

This section is self-explanatory, just follow the example.

HOBBY GOALS

Define some hobbies, activities you want to learn or do.

RELATIONSHIP GOALS

What kind of relationships do you want to create? For example, do you want to find a lifelong mate, or a girlfriend? Define what kind of a person you want them to be in character, personality, physical attributes, intelligence, tastes in food, lifestyle, etc.

Everyone has dreams, but in many cases they don't believe they will actually happen. I want you to shift your thinking to believing you create your reality. Define the main dream you would like to see fulfilled in the next couple of years or so.

WHAT I KNOW ABOUT MY LIFE AND MYSELF

This section deals with you being aware of the important aspects of your life.

First, define what kind of understanding you want to have about the spiritual aspect of your life. Whether you have a faith of some kind? Do you believe in the afterlife? This section's intent is not to indoctrinate you, but to have you define what you believe spiritually about your life and your purpose for being on the planet. This will allow you to have meaning in why you do the things you do in your life and give you a greater sense of purpose.

Secondly, under the emotional section, define what you want to learn about your emotions. Which ones are dominant in your life and which ones do you want to experience the most? If there are too many negative emotions happening, then you may want that to change to have more positive emotions rule your life and your day. One of the concepts I have taken from leadership training is that in order for us to become successful in anything, we need to take 100% responsibility for our life and all that happens to us. Take responsibility for your own emotions and make adjustments to the kind of emotions you want to experience more in your day.

RELATIONSHIPS WITH PEOPLE IN YOUR LIFE

This section is probably one of the most important areas to plan because the way we respond to others is, in most cases, the way others will respond to us. Here, you define the kind of relationship you want to have with various groups of people in your life.

How do you want to be with family members? For example, with your mother; do you want to have a deeper relationship with her, get to know her history better, etc.? How do you want to be with your business associates or colleagues at work? Do you want an honest relationship that is non-competitive in nature, be able to have a trusting relationship based on mutual respect? With acquaintances or people you know briefly, you may still want to have a policy where you always look for the "gold" in people when you meet them. For this section, it is enough to just describe in a sentence or two what you want to create.

HOW WOULD YOU LIKE PEOPLE TO THINK OF YOU?

How would you like to be perceived by others? It's a hard question at times to ask ourselves. However, if we want to grow as a person of quality, a character that others want to be around and respect, we also must become the kind of person deserving of such respect.

In many cases, what we view ourselves as is not what others see. This is something that takes five minutes to learn, but a lifetime to master.

WHAT SPECIFICALLY WOULD YOU LIKE TO LEARN DURING YOUR LIFE?

We all look at our lives at some point and think about the lessons we learned that helped us grow, mend a broken friendship, or move forward in our life. It's important to assess what we have learned so we can assess what we may still have to learn. It may be something like getting better at expressing our feelings to loved ones, learning to say no to people or realizing we need to change the way we think to produce different results. One of the main areas I believe we all need to learn from is our relationships with people. If a relationship is valuable in our life, it's because we learn something from that relationship. It's good to define what you want to learn, in your relationships as a spouse, friend, leader, etc. Then you actually will intentionally be motivated to grow in those relationships.

The final part of this plan helps you define roughly how much money you need to earn a year or have in savings or in investments to allow you to live the life according to your life plan. Take the time to actually do this because it will force you to make this more real and increase your faith that it can happen! This life plan defines the dream you want to live while on earth. We all want to be successful and we are happy when we are pursuing our dreams. This definition of success is worth remembering: "Success is the progressive realization of a worthwhile dream."[19]

Life Plan Template

WHAT DO I VALUE? (EXAMPLES)

I value the feeling and the belief that I can go all out and towards the dreams and desires of my heart without feeling guilty, doubtful, fearful, inferior and ashamed.

I value making the most of my time, getting closer to goals I have set for my life each day.

I value maintaining my optimal physical health, vitality and energy.

I value looking strong, beautiful outside and inside, brimming with health and energy, mastering my emotions so that when negative things happen to me, I can respond peacefully, calmly, wisely and still be on track to my given tasks and commitments.

I value being around friends, people that also feel and think about life the way I do.

I value living my day to the fullest, meeting all my tasks each day with a healthy, positive attitude so that others may also be impacted in a positive, encouraging way!

I value the opportunity to always learn something new about people and about myself each day, so that I can be that much wiser, perfected in character and able to deal positively and nurturing with others and myself.

I value the opportunity to build healthy relationships with friends, acquaintances, clients, business associates, and with my loved ones.

I value times where I can enjoy life, good weather, good healthy food and function in my healthy, fit body!

WHAT MY LIFE WILL LOOK LIKE:

Financially in the near future: (Eight-accounts method of budgeting)

(Example) "I will have all my debts paid in two years and have enough saved to put a down payment of at least 50% on a townhouse in the suburb of Ottawa."

Socially in the next 30 days, two months or three months:

(Example) "I will be socially wise and able to develop healthier working relationships with a select few at work who feed my life with positive feedback, but don't allow the others who are negative in their attitude to taint my space with their gossip, complaining, etc."

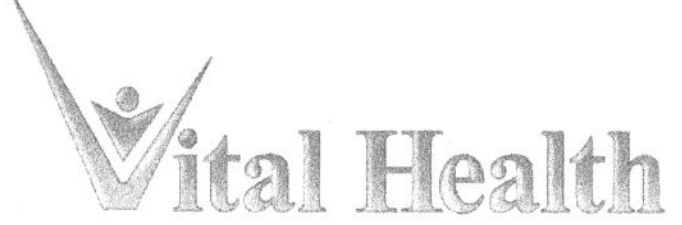

Emotionally immediately, from now on:

(Example) "I will catch myself whenever I find myself feeling sorry for myself about a past hurt that someone did to me, and replace it with things that I can be thankful for and good things that are happening to me in my life that I can focus on as a blessing. Have an attitude of gratitude for all the good things in my life so far."

Physically in three months, two months or one month, try to set a time line here:

(Example) "My body-fat will have decreased significantly, lose about two inches in the waist and be able to power-walk, jog 3.5 km three times a week on a regular basis, workout for at least 30-45 minutes at the gym three times a week no matter what my schedule is like..."

At Work or in My Business:

(Example) "I will only have to work 30 hours a week, but still do the same amount of work and make double the income..."

What Kind of Experiences You Want to Have:

At Work:
(Example) "I will try to communicate better so there is less misunderstanding with my manager"

At Home:
(Example) "Be less busy, more organized with my chores so I will have more leisure time to relax and do those personal growth activities like reading, writing letters to friends and trying new healthy recipes"

At the Gym:

(Example) "Talk less and focus on my workouts more and be done on time"

At Social Gatherings with Friends:

(Example) "Have a more laid-back approach, listen to what's going on more to my friends' lives; show more interest in what concerns them..."

Your Special Self-Nurture time, i.e. jog, bike ride or walks:

(Example) "Let go of all my worries for the day during the jog or walk and focus on just the breathing and the moment-to-moment surroundings and all the beauty that is around me in sight and sounds..."

During My Groceries, Errands & Chores:

(Example) "Show more appreciation to the clerks, cashiers and sales people for the work they do and smile to everyone when they cross my path, just so they feel better from the quick exchange"

If you had all the money that you could ever want, how would you live each day or week starting from the moment you awaken to the time you go to bed?

(Example) "...I would do my morning floor exercises for 10 minutes and have about half an hour for my shower and bathroom routine. Then I would have about an hour to make a healthy, delicious breakfast, make my healthy lunch and have a half hour to sit and eat it peacefully, take my supplements without being anxious about anything. Then I would walk to work and take in the sights, along the way. I would work at my job only every other day, during the week

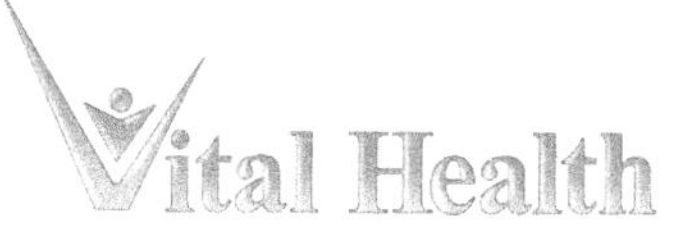

for about eight hours and on Tuesdays and Thursdays, go for my long 10-km jogs, then have lunch with friends at a restaurant of our choosing that serves healthy gourmet cuisine, etc..."

Personal Goals:

Leisure Goals

(Example) "Save enough to go down south with the whole family for a week"

Activity, Interest or Hobby Goals

(Example) "Learn how to Salsa with a partner without missing a step..."

Relationship Goals

(Example) "Fly overseas to see relatives for about two weeks"

Main Big Dream

(Example) "I want to be able to live in a house that truly nurtures health and well-being as people function inside. There will be lots of windows, high ceilings, stain-glass skylights with stone brick walls, hardwood floors, woodstove, fireplace and a cold cellar to store vegetables."

What I Know About My Life and Myself

Spiritually

(Example) "I will have a deeper and a more clear understanding of the Divine purpose of why I have been directed in this career path the last 10 years..."

In Terms of My Emotions

(Example) "I want to be more aware of how I handle certain emotions in my life like sadness, anger and worry. I want to know what triggers my sad feelings during the week..."

Relationships with People in Your Life?

Business Associates

My Family

Member's Names:

Acquaintances

Fellow Staff

Community Members (Doctors, bus drivers, teachers, etc.)

With My Friends

How Do I Want To Be With My:

Close Friends

New Friends

Acquaintances (Dentists, receptionists, manager at the club, etc.)

How Would You Like People To Think of You?

(Example) I would like others to think of me as someone who has...

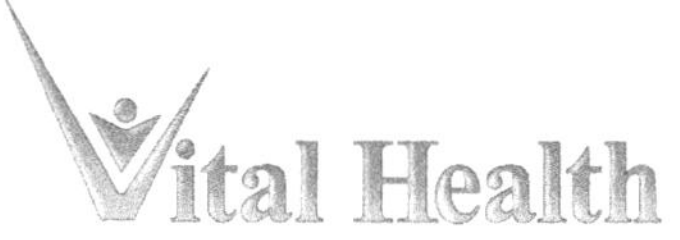

What Specifically Would I Like to Learn During My Life?

Spiritually

(Example) "I would like to learn how to live each day full of joy and contentment even in the midst of pressure, adversity, conflict and fear."

Physically

(Example) "I would like to experience peak health, vitality, energy, endurance and well-developed lean physique. Also have full mastery of eye, hand coordination. Balance, speed, flexibility and power through the expression of martial arts, sparring, aerobic exercise classes, running, track & field drills, plyometrics and body building."

Relationships

(Example) "I would like to learn how to be a true friend to..."

Financially

(Example) "I will make myself financially free and successful through..."

Technically

(Example) "I would like to know the technical skill of designing a website, etc..."

How Much Money I Will Need to Do the Things I Want to According to this Life Plan?

(Example) "I am going to need at least (Dollar Value) etc..."

Healthy Thinking for Life

I want to help you reflect on the deep reasons why you want to make lifestyle changes. If you don't define clearly "why" you do something, then usually the commitment can flounder. Unfortunately, most people live their lives not being committed to anything and end up going through life a "wondering generality".[20] Define how you feel about yourself. Go deep in your heart. Do you feel you deserve to be beautiful, brilliant and successful? I'm asking this because many of us did not get positive encouragement in the early part of our lives. We were often told what we could not do, and to be realistic about our goals. As we grew up, we came to accept that some of our goals were "pipe dreams" or unrealistic, or something that others would achieve, not us; ideas such as becoming a millionaire or getting in amazing shape. But in reality, you can be, do, or have anything you really want if you are willing to increase your belief and "GO For IT"! I am here to tell you that. Consider answering the questions on the next page, Healthy Thinking for Life, and try to be as honest as you can with your answers.

WRITE DOWN FIVE LIFE CHANGES.

These will be made within the next 12 weeks and will help with the progress to your healthier lifestyle. They are called Life Changes, and not goals, because most people default to earlier lifestyle habits after reaching a goal. Life Changes gives the intention of a permanent shift in your lifestyle. It could be something as simple as no more lattes at lunch; instead, you are going to try different herbal teas.

IDENTIFY THREE PATTERNS OF ACTION.

Which actions have been sabotaging your success? A sabotaging action could be saying yes to dessert when you are out with friends. What if, instead, you had fruit or found an organic bakery where desserts are sweetened with honey or maple syrup? That would become an action that would make you stronger in your stand on how you want to eat when you go out with friends. What about deciding to start shopping at the health food store for some of your produce, so you are surrounded by healthier people and attitudes? A Pattern of Action can help you identify your pitfalls, but also direct you to achieving your Life Changes.

Life Change Decisions

THE REASONS FOR MAKING THE DECISION TO CHANGE:

How do I feel deep down inside?

How do I feel about myself?

Am I confident, energetic and strong?

Do I often wonder if I'm on the right path?

What are the pros and cons of continuing in the direction I'm going?

Would I like to create a brighter future?

For me to be pleased with the progress in my life and my body, the five most important Life Changes I need to make within the next 12 weeks are:

1.

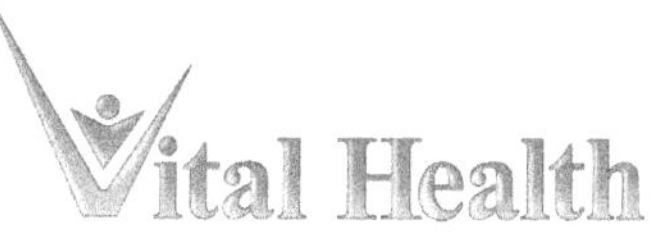

2.

3.

4.

5.

Three patterns of action that may hold me back are:

1.

2.

3.

Three patterns of action that will help me reach my Life Change Decisions are:

1.

2.

3.

About Body Measurements

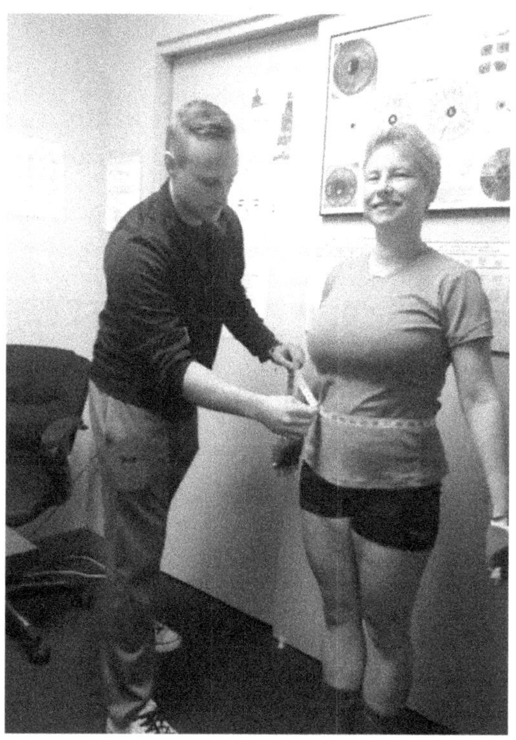

If you are trying to make changes to your body shape, you will want to take measurements; starting weight, body fat percentage, resting heart rate, resting blood pressure and body circumference measurements. By taking measurements each month or every three months you will see how many inches you have lost in different areas of your body. Numbers on paper will give you positive reinforcement to stick to a weight-loss or muscle-building program. The numbers will tell you if you are making progress or hitting a plateau.

Weight: Weight scales can be deceiving. I discourage my clients from focusing too much on the scales. Muscle weighs twice as much as fat and when you are exercising as well as following a weight-loss eating plan, you may gain lean muscle and lose fat at the same time. Your weight may not change much on the scale, but your body-fat percentage may be lower.

As you progress on your program, a better indicator of weight loss will be the way your clothes fit and the way you look in the mirror. You may notice clothing looser in areas where you are losing fat. Areas of your body that are developing from the exercising will appear and feel tighter, harder, and more defined. Some areas will be more noticeable than others, depending on how much outer fat layer you have. Someone who is leaner will show body development sooner because of the thinner layer of fat covering their muscles.

Body fat: You can get your body fat percentage measured in different ways. An instructor at your local health club can measure body fat percentage for you or you can buy an electronic weight scale that will also calculate your body fat. As long as you can get an approximate number within a few percentages, that will do. A healthy fat percentage for females can be around 12 to 17 percent. In many health charts, that number is often 20 percent and higher.[21] However, I believe women can easily be lower than 17 percent and be very healthy.

Resting heart rate: For the average person who is not an athlete or physically active, this is usually around 65 to 72 bpm (beats per minute). If you run or jog regularly, play a sport such as soccer, cross-country ski, participate in aerobic classes or any other type of activity that increases the heart rate for a sustained period of time, then your resting heart rate may be significantly lower. It may be around 55 to 65 bpm. Elite runners have resting heart rates as low as 48 bpm. Their heart is so strong it does not need to pump as much with the same amount of blood throughout their body. The heart works less. Some people may genetically have a low heart rate. It is good to check your blood pressure to make sure it's not too high or too low. The normal range should be around 120/80, 115/75, 125/85, etc. If your heart rate is extremely low or high, then you need to consult your doctor. He or she needs to know about your plan to start exercise training along with a healthy eating plan so they can advise you of any necessary precautions.

Body circumference measurements: When measuring the arms, wrap the tape around the bicep portion of your arm while holding it straight out to the side. Then place the tape around both shoulders. For the chest, wrap the tape around the nipple line. To measure the waist, find the narrowest point above the hips. For the buttocks, place the tape around the highest point of the buttocks, which is also your hip area. For the thighs, wrap the tape around the middle of the thigh and do the same for the calf. In most cases, I only measure one side of the body, but you may want to know what your measurements are on both sides.

How often to measure: Try not to measure too often. Give your body at least a month to show changes. Do not get discouraged if you do not see a significant weight drop exactly in a week, just keep to the weight-loss meal program as shown in the book and you will see the changes. The weight never drops evenly. You may not see any changes, then in a week or two you may drop two pounds or more. For a healthy weight-loss program, it's best to have an average of a pound lost per week.

For those who want to gain: Weight gain in muscle size may be a slower process, but be patient. Stick to the mass gaining meal program and do not over-train or do too much cardio. You end up burning too many calories which will be counterproductive in you gaining some weight and muscle. Your weight gain will not just be muscle, but a percentage of the gain will also be in fat, water with the muscle. In most cases unless you are genetically endowed with a very lean body, you will need to keep your body fat percentage up around at least 12 percent to gain mass easily if you are gaining muscle naturally.

Note your achievements: In the achievement section, record the dates when you lost so many pounds or gained an inch on your arms. This is a very concrete way of recording your successes. So when you feel down about your progress, you can look at your achievements to encourage yourself that results are on their way. In the comment section, write out things you may have learned about how your body loses weight the best. Maybe you noticed when you stopped eating those snacks after 8 pm the weight came off faster that week. These records of your progress will help you better understand how your body works when it comes to weight loss or weight or muscle gain.

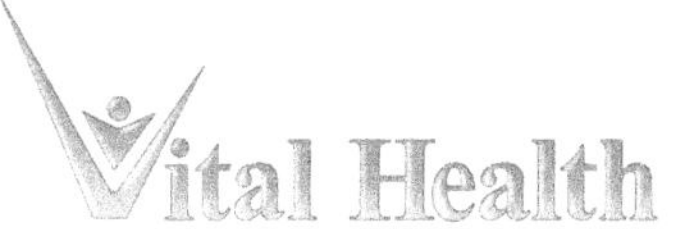

BODY MEASUREMENTS

	Date:	Date:	Date:
Body Weight in lbs			
Body Fat %			
Resting Heart Rate			
Resting Blood Pressure			

MEASUREMENTS IN INCHES

Upper Arms	Left:	Right:	Left:	Right:	Left:	Right:
Shoulders						
Chest						
Waist						
Buttocks/Hips						
Thighs	Left:	Right:	Left:	Right:	Left:	Right:
Calves	Left:	Right:	Left:	Right:	Left:	Right:

Achievements:

Comments:

About Lifestyle Habits & Behaviour

The following questionnaire will help you assess your lifestyle and become aware of your lifestyle habits. You can start to make changes in those habits that are not helping you in becoming healthier or fit.

For example, if you are working more than 60 hours, six days a week, that may be one of the reasons you feel highly stressed. Your body is not getting enough rest and recuperative time. It you smoke, you need to seriously look at stopping because it ages your body, not to mention the risks of developing respiratory diseases and cancer of the throat, mouth and lungs. Alcohol in small doses on a weekend with dinner is not a concern; however, every night after dinner where there are two to three glasses can have negative health effects.[22] In regards to coffee and tea, keep it to one 8 oz. cup a day if you cannot stop having it daily. Coffee is one of the highest sprayed plants that we consume. Ideally, I would choose organic, naturally decaffeinated coffee which still has about 4% caffeine – enough to still give you a boost. Consider your sleep patterns. Are you getting an average of eight hours of uninterrupted sleep where enough of the hormone Melatonin can be produced? This hormone gives you energy, increases the immune system, enhances libido and has anti-aging effects. Is your energy high in the morning, then you crash mid-afternoon? This may be because you are eating too much empty high-sugar foods, like boxed cereals and sweetened coffee, which causes extreme highs and lows of energy from the Insulin spikes. To remedy this, consume eggs with vegetables for breakfast and maybe a protein shake with omega

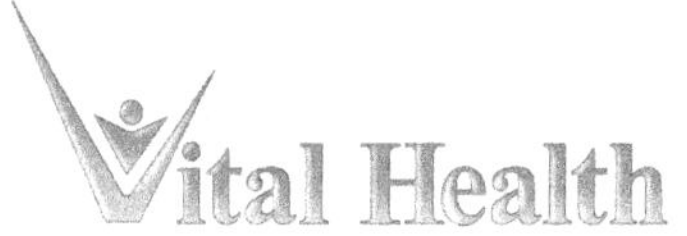

oils with your coffee. This will cause a slow release of sugar throughout the day as these foods digest slower and enter the blood stream slowly, giving you sustained energy throughout the day.

The Nutritional Background section of the questionnaire will help you identify what you consume each day. You can see which foods may be causing high sugar spikes and weight gain and which foods are processed and need to be replaced with healthier, natural choices. When you list your favourite foods, realize there is usually a healthier option. For example, instead of ice-cream, try a soy-based frozen dessert or locally made gelato which is free of commercial preservatives and uses less sugar, often sweetened with fruit or raw cane sugar.

LIFESTYLE HABITS & BEHAVIOUR QUESTIONNAIRE

Occupation ____________________ Description of work Performed _________________________

Hours worked per week _____________ Number of Days worked Per Week___________________

Are there any other major "stressors" in your life?____

Have you ever smoked? *Yes/No/Currently;*

How long have you smoked? _____________________ # of cigarettes per day? ________________

Do you drink Alcohol? *Yes/No/Currently*; # of drinks per week ___________

Do you drink Coffee/Tea *Yes/No/Currently*; # of cups per day? ___________

How do you consider your sleep patterns? *Good/Average/Poor*

How many hours do you sleep per night? _____________________

Energy Levels in the...

Morning *Good/Average/Poor*

Afternoon *Good/Average/Poor*

Night *Good/Average/Poor*

NUTRITIONAL BACKGROUND:

How many of the following meals and what foods do you typically eat daily?

Breakfast *Yes/No* ____

Mid Morning Snack *Yes/No* ____

Lunch *Yes/No* ____

Mid Afternoon Snack *Yes/No* ____

Dinner *Yes/No* ____

Evening Snack *Yes/No* ____

Late Night Snack *Yes/No* ____

Other *Yes/No* ____

List your favorite foods: ____

Gain Muscle to Lose Weight

Sarcopenia is a condition of extreme muscle loss, occurring especially in people as they age and become less active. The result of this condition is osteoporosis. In order to keep bones strong, muscles need to contract. Dr. William Evans, director of nutrition and metabolism at University of Arkansas for Medical Sciences discovered that many of the elderly in nursing homes were not there because of cognitive impairment or disease, but mainly because of muscle weakness. Studies done in 1990 presented in the *Journal of the American Medical Association* showed muscle mass and strength of 90-year-old subjects was greatly improved in as little as eight weeks through resistance training.[23] Along with the nutritional changes you will be learning in this book, I strongly suggest you also start a basic exercise program at home or at a gym. If you want to learn more, I suggest you view my exercise videos on my website. If you feel you need more personal guidance, then hiring a personal trainer at your local gym is a great investment where you will really accelerate your learning and progress.

The best way to lose weight and keep it off is to increase your metabolism through training with weights which increases muscle mass, a good balanced protein, carbohydrate and fat meal plan. Please ignore all your fears about getting too bulked up with muscle from weight training! That is a total myth! It actually is very difficult to gain pure lean muscle and keep it on. It takes consistent work. It will actually cause you to have a leaner, more sculpted hard body which is what you should have when you are healthy and fit.

Most people think they have to do as much cardiovascular training as possible to lose weight. With cardio, you may get an extra 40-80 calories burned after a moderate session based upon the level of intensity and duration. In order to burn a large amount of calories after aerobic activity you would have to do it for a long period of time, typically an hour and a half or two. [24] Not everybody can sustain such long cardio regiments in their daily schedules, so combining about 30 minutes of cardio with about 30 minutes of weight and floor exercises is realistic for most people. Do that four to five times a week if you are trying to shed excess fat off the body fast. If you are on a more moderate program, then three times a week with a fairly strict regiment on the eating plan. "Studies have demonstrated that after a weight training workout, the metabolism can be boosted for up to 36 hours post-workout, meaning rather than burning say 60 calories an hour while sitting and watching TV, you're burning 70. While you may think, 'Big deal - 10 extra calories', when you multiply this by 36 hours, you can see what a huge difference that makes in your daily calorie expenditure over that day and a half."[25]

While cardiovascular training will help burn calories, it does not provide a long-term metabolic boost. Increasing the amount of muscle in your body is the most effective way to lose those unwanted pounds. Also eating foods that have the right nutrients to nourish your body so it will grow in strength and endurance to meet the demands of your training regime is very important. This is why I always stress that people consume enough clean protein to help gain enough lean muscle as they train in the gym with some sort of resistance-based exercise along with stretching, yoga, cross-fit style training and various aerobic type exercises.

IMPORTANCE OF PROTEIN

Protein is the building block for muscle growth and a whole lot of other material the body needs to repair, grow and rebuild. It makes up about 17% of the body in the form of its tissue structures, cell membranes and genetic material. All proteins have a function in the body. There is no storage of protein like there is for fat

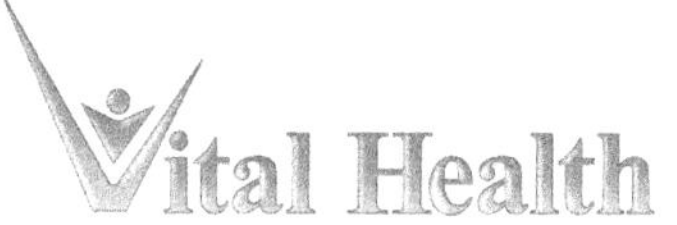

in the body. The protein in the body can be classified into three main functional groups which is:

Muscle Protein

Visceral (abdominal organs) protein

Plasma proteins and plasma amino acids [26]

Recovery of protein synthesis occurs during the following four to eight hours, up to 48 hours after exercise. Therefore post-exercise intake of carbohydrates and protein is important to maximize protein synthesis in the muscle and for its recovery. [27]

This is why in many cases adding some vegetable based or whey based protein to the meal plan is a good option for many people so the lean muscle development will happen more readily and their recovery will be better as well from their training at the gym. I am not going to address all the controversy of using whey protein verses rice, pea protein, etc. For the purposes of this book, as long as you are getting extra protein supplementation from quality sources, then you will benefit. Read the labels of your protein and meal replacement products and make sure there are not too many sugars, sugar substitutes and preservatives like fructose, corn syrup, maltose, sucrose, sucralose, and aspartame. Try to use non-flavoured, good quality whey isolate and mix it with fresh fruit for flavour. Brown rice, pea protein, hemp and egg protein are good choices as well.

For people who are trying to lose fat and excess weight, here are some facts about how lean muscle gain affects weight-loss.

It is estimated that just one pound of muscle will burn an extra 35 to 50 calories per day, at rest. That means extra calories are being burnt off while you are relaxing, at work and even sleeping! An extra 10 pounds of muscle will therefore burn approximately 350 to 500 extra calories per day, or over 3,500 per week. In order to lose one pound of fat you must burn an extra 3,500 calories. This means that if you increase the amount of muscle mass in your body by 10 pounds, you will lose a pound of fat every 7 to 10 days, without making any other changes!

About Positive Statements and Empowering Questions

When you become serious about making changes to your lifestyle to become healthier, to improve your nutrition and to make exercising a way of life, you will need to have a philosophy of what kind of person you want to be! Your beliefs about who you are as you live this life as a human being needs to be clear or you can easily be distracted or give up when the "going" gets tough. You need to realize that you have to change the way you view or think about life because usually that is what has caused most people to end up in a toxic lifestyle, eating on the run and ending up in a high stress lifestyle that has resulted in them becoming overweight and undernourished. Unfortunately, we have become a very consumer-oriented society where people spend a lot of their energies on obtaining material goods to satisfy their need to have things. Not that having nice things is wrong. But, in many cases, life is out of balance.

Many people do not take enough time to enjoy their own company. I believe many people are unhappy with their self-image and may be in partial denial of it. One of the ways you can feel more comfortable with who you are is by learning to make the journey inward to know who you are as a spiritual being.

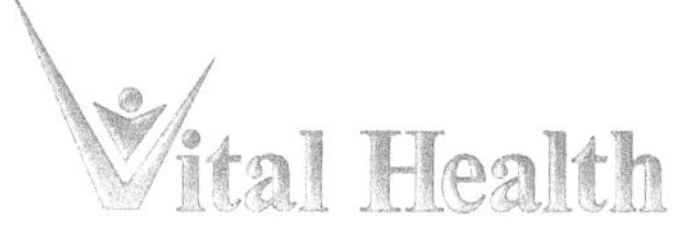

SEPARATING FROM THE MIND

Eckhart Tolle in *The Power of Now* warns against identifying yourself with your mind. When you think you are your mind, then you operate from a place of fear and want and this is where dysfunctions occur. You end up living out of your "ego" where it feels vulnerable and threatened so it attaches itself to the problems in your life. This is why so many people's sense of self is connected to their problems. This leads to people having a lot of difficulty in letting go of their problems because that would mean a loss of their self-identity, because there has been so much investment into their pain and suffering.[28] This is one of the reasons why so many people have a hard time sticking to an exercise regiment and taking the time to cook healthy meals. To make healthier meals usually takes longer in preparation, hence you have more time to be reflective. When you walk in the park for 45 minutes, it causes you to face your sense of self. This is uncomfortable to many people because they have to start looking at who they are inside and deal with their fears and pain. However, it is a good way to re-invent yourself and make the changes in your thinking so you become a more empowered individual.

MEDITATIVE BREATHING

Another way to connect more with the body, and not the mind, is through meditative breathing (similar to *pranayama* breathing) – taking deep breaths through the nostrils and blowing out slowly through the mouth. Many believe this breathing allows "The Life Force" to enter more into our being to bring healing and restoration at all levels.[29] This is a practice I now do on a regular basis. Close your eyes so you are less distracted and count as you inhale/exhale and do at least 35 breaths first thing in the morning. It takes about eight minutes. On days where you have more time, increase to 50 or 60 breaths. This allows you to relax the body and decrease anxiety. I even practice this when I am driving and I feel stressed – but do keep your eyes open when driving. This is one of the main ways

I physically decrease feelings of stress in my life that I may be experiencing at any given moment.[30]

POSITIVE STATEMENTS AND AFFIRMATIONS

Another motivation tool that will make a difference, even though it may seem subtle, is to write out positive statements and affirmations. These will help us focus on the goals we have made for ourselves. Look at these statements and affirmations regularly so they become a part of everyday thinking. I believe by speaking positive affirmative words on a daily basis, or multiple times a day, it will fill us, as Norman Vincent Peale points out, with thoughts of faith, confidence and security. This will force out any doubtful thoughts about succeeding in this new weight-loss eating plan and fitness program. [31] And when we speak, that energy vibrates through our bones and has a physical affect on our body and our brain.

Here is a positive affirmation sheet you can post on a bedroom or bathroom wall to look at everyday. Read it quickly as you get out of the shower or brush your teeth. If you look at a few sentences and rehearse them, this will help get them into your subconscious. You will start to be more aware of how you think about yourself and about those commitments to go for that walk or jog or get in that planned workout, even in the midst of social engagements and job tasks. Ideally, read positive affirmations aloud at the beginning of your day. Aim for once throughly for at least 31 days because after 31 days, it can become a habit. Remember you have to win the battle in your mind before you can win it physically!

POSITIVE STATEMENTS AND EMPOWERING QUESTIONS

(Say one of these statements every day!)

- How can I lose fat and enjoy the process?

- What can I do today that will help me get closer to my weight loss goal?
- What can I eat right now at this meal that will help me lose body fat?
- How great am I going to feel after I finish my workout today?
- My metabolism is getting faster every day.
- I am getting leaner every day.
- I like the way I look.
- I am 100% responsible for my results.
- Whatever it takes, I'll do it.
- I like eating healthy foods.
- I love working out.
- Training early in the morning is exhilarating.
- I have time for anything I am committed to.
- I like myself.
- I can do it.
- I'll do it.

GETTING THE GUT IN ORDER

I believe the only real way to truly get your body healthy is to have healthy digestion and maintain it. To have a healthy functioning digestive system, we need to do the following:

Reduce inflammation in the body and the intestine caused by different food allergies

Improve absorption by increasing enzymes and restoring the correct acid levels

Establish a healthy good bacterial level in the digestive tract

Repair and heal the intestinal wall, balancing the main hormones that control fat-burn, sugar levels, weight-loss, hunger, energy, stress and rejuvenating sleep, etc.

Reduce the damaging effects of stress on the bowels

The digestive system is controlled by the hormonal system which is controlled by the central nervous system (CNS), made up of the brain and spine.

However, there is also the enteric nervous system (ENS) which runs the length of the whole intestinal tract. It allows communication between the nerve cells of the digestive tract to muscles, glands and vessels. There is almost as many neurotransmitters in the digestive area as there are in the brain in addition to the major cells of the immune system. This is why the digestive system can carry out its various functions without our conscious effort. This is also why we experience pain, heartburn, gas or diarrhea because our digestion is letting us know something is not right in our system. Therefore, when we are not eating the right foods at the right time it creates stress on our system. However, external stress from our environment or our own feelings and emotions can have profound effects on our digestive system as well, since we have this "gut" brain in our system.

This is why I have introduced the Life Plan exercise, along with the other positive mental building exercise tools. The Life Plan will help you clarify internal conflicts you may be experiencing. These exercises will help you build a more harmonious life. If there are unresolved anger, bitterness, resentment, fear, and un-forgiveness in your heart, I strongly encourage you to get counselling or help in becoming free of those negative emotions. If not, these emotions can have a negative effect on your digestion.[32] Meditative breathing, discussed above, can be helpful with ridding yourself of these emotions negatively affecting digestion.

Medications are another factor that can affect your inner awareness of your emotions, your mental state and your varied internal physiological systems. This is especially true when you are dependent on their use. I believe our brain is a transmitter and receiver of frequencies from our external environment, which includes other brains. Medications will short-circuit our frequencies so that we are not clearly connected to an inner guidance of awareness; what is going on in our mind and life. When we are "numb", we are more susceptible to following other people's influence instead of our own thinking. A good example of this is the millions of people in North America dependent on medications that doctors prescribe instead of taking control of their own health and healing the body before the medications become necessary to live.

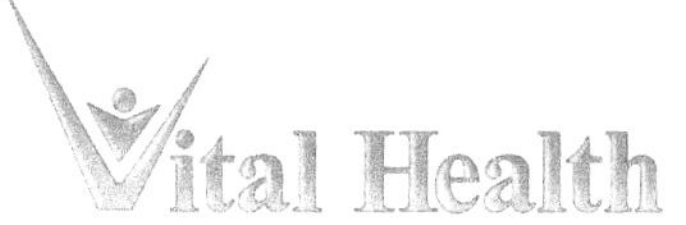

INTESTINAL CLEANSE

Before we get into the Vital Health System of healthy meal plans to lean up or gain muscle or lose weight, I suggest people first go through a bowel (intestinal) cleanse, parasite cleanse, kidney cleanse, liver flush and heavy metal cleanse as prescribed in my Inner Cleanse Program. The incredible amount of concentrated micro-nutrients in raw vegetables and fruit juices actually helps restore a weakened immune system. Follow the cleanse protocol in the order given as much as possible. For instance, if you do the liver flush before the kidney cleanse – depending on how much toxins you have – you may feel sick and have a stronger reaction. You will find that after the cleanse, a lot of hormonal imbalance and health issues will decrease, if not be entirely gone. Many of the symptoms people struggle with, such as acid indigestion, bloating, constipation, gas, fatigue, and mental fogginess, disappear after the program.

Let's start with the Cleansing Meal Program Level 2.

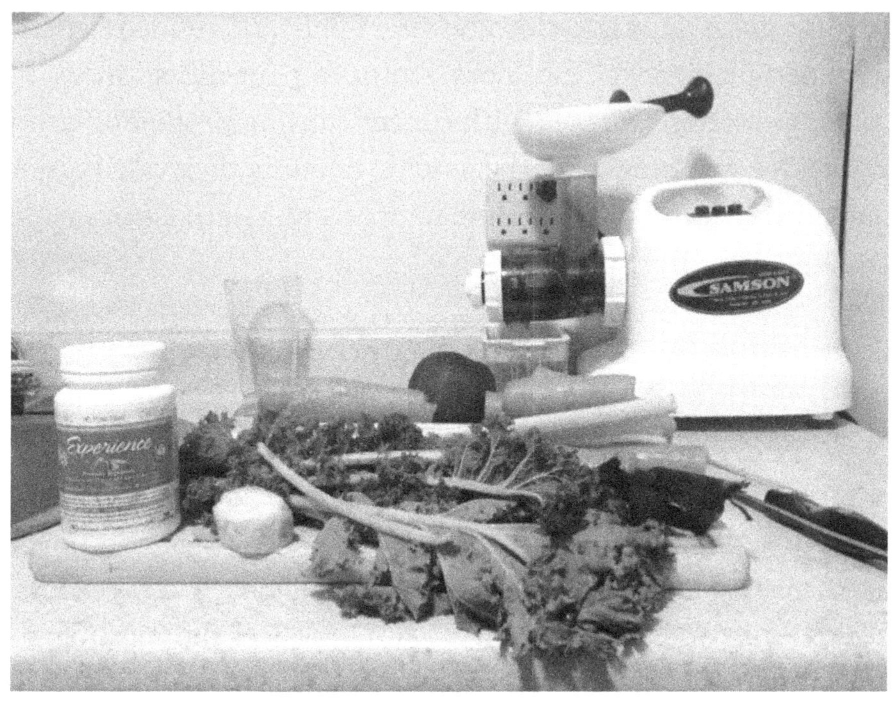

Cleansing

WHY CLEANSE?

Based on the amount of processed foods we eat, most of us who live in the West need to cleanse our digestive system every few years or every year. This is because the majority of the western population does not eat a sufficient diet of organic, raw vegetables, whole grains, etc. Most of us consume processed foods which usually contain toxins, preservatives, food colouring, fillers and refined sugars[33]. White flour and refined foods are a huge contributor to poor digestion in the bowels. Non-organic produce are sprayed with cancer-causing pesticides, synthetic fertilizers, herbicides, and fungicides that end up in our bodies, causing a toxic state that can lead to diseases, hormonal imbalances and health issues.

EXCESS ESTROGEN

An example of this is the effect growth hormones and antibiotics fed to livestock, poultry and dairy animals have on our bodies. Excess estrogen hormone levels can occur as we consume animal products not naturally raised. This excess estrogen leads to weight gain or excess fat which again produces more estrogen from the fat cells. The progressive weight gain from this leads to insulin resistance which increases the risk of estrogen dominance as explained by Dr. Natasha Turner in her book *The Hormone Diet.* There are many contributing factors that cause estrogen dominance. First, high stress levels cause the body to respond by producing cortisol from progesterone, leaving an excess of estrogen. Second, xenoestrogens that mimic estrogen are compounds found in dairy, beef, pesticides, herbicides, plastics and cosmetics. Third, impaired liver function due to too much alcohol, drug use, and fatty liver and different forms of liver disease can cause excess estrogen. Fourthly, weak digestion from low dietary fibre and weak bacterial balance in the intestine can hinder the proper elimination of estrogen from the body. Fifth cause is from a high consumption of saturated and polyunsaturated fats which increase estrogen production. Sixth cause is when the diet is deficient in zinc, magnesium, and vitamin B6.[34]In addition to this list, deficiencies in omega-3 foods, such as fermented cod liver oil, choline, calcium, iodine, selenium and vitamin D, can also bring on the estrogen buildup.[35]

During a cleanse, the foods you want to stay away from are all dairy products, all grains, corn in various forms, hydrogenated oils, alcohol, caffeine, peanuts and peanut-containing products, sugar and artificial sweeteners, all citrus fruits (except lemons), red meats, pork, beef, lamb, cold cuts, bacon and every kind of sausage.

HOW THE BODY BECOMES TOXIC

There are many digestive consequences of the average diet in North America. The transit time of food becomes extremely slow and, in many cases, people are constipated or have incomplete elimination issues with undigested fecal matter in the colon wall and encrusted mucus buildup along the small intestinal wall. The nutrient content of the food is low due to processing and overcooking. Unlike raw vegetables and fruits, which have lots of fibre material that sweeps away buildup in the colon wall, the low water content of many dry processed foods, which includes most bread products, does not allow the intestinal wall to get cleaned. Instead, the digestive organs such as your liver, kidneys and small intestine are weakened so they cannot carry out the clean-up process necessary to get rid of toxic buildup in the system. These organs are the body's natural cleaning team and when they are working at optimal level, they can get rid of the toxin compounds in the body.[36]Eventually, people end up with an extra film coating made up of excess mucus mixed with undigested food residue which eventually becomes an extra layer of toxic film along the walls of the intestine. This is known as mucoid plaque. From a prolonged cleanse of the body or a strict juice cleanse of five days or more, you can pass some of this mucoid plaque in a rope-like fashion when you eliminate. I personally experienced this. I did a strict juice cleanse with no solid food for about five days. I passed what seemed like a short length of almost black stool that looked like rope. After that, I felt amazing. Even though at the time I was doing a semi-fast cleansing program, where I still ate some raw vegetables with juices and ate some fish or chicken every two days for almost 35 days, I still passed more toxic waste out of my body. When people consume regularly a lot of white flour foods, pastas, greasy, deep-fried breaded foods and little vegetables, it can lead to slower transit time, constipation because of the low water content in these types of foods. If changes in eating habits are not made, various bowel diseases like diverticulitis, polyps, leaky gut syndrome, IBS, and other bowel issues can result. One way to help digest foods like breads, pastas with meat sauce and breaded foods is to take an extra glass of fresh raw vegetable juice, extra probiotics and enzyme supplements in capsules. This way you help the body with the enzymes, the good bacteria and the juice from the raw vegetables, the fibre and the water content of these foods to help breakdown and digest the heavy flour and high fat content meal.

ENZYMES

Enzymes are protein-like substances formed in plants and in animals. They act as catalysts in chemical reactions in the body. They help speed up processes in the body, especially in the digestive processes that occur as food is broken down to assimilate into the cells of our body. Glands and organs depend upon enzymatic activity and cannot function without them. There are 700 enzymes that work in the body and each has a particular function. If the body is missing one of these enzymes, there is a risk of a health issue. These enzymes can only be obtained from raw, living foods which is why when you consume enough raw foods you have more energy. The enzymes from the food provide the energy! When the enzymes are missing it causes the body to over-work the glands to produce the missing enzymes which leads to the glands being out of balance in their hormonal secretions, which leads to you feeling tired. This is why people who eat too much cooked foods and not enough raw foods have little energy.[37]

UNHEALTHY MUCUS AND NORMAL MUCUS

Many of the foods such as animal protein, chocolate, dairy products, and processed foods made from white flour and deep-fried foods, such as French fries, which are cooked in processed oils, causes our digestive system to become more acidic and toxic. Hence the mucus in our body becomes dirtier. This excess toxic mucus builds up over time into what is known as mucoid plaque which then builds up along the intestinal wall.[38] Normal mucus in the body is clear and protects the surface membranes of the body. It engulfs anything we consume into the body. However, when we ingest foods that contain toxins, the mucus becomes sticky, cloudy and thicker. Over time, this excess thick mucus also traps fecal material and other debris which creates an environment that is quite acidic and promotes growth of negative microforms (parasites). Furthermore, stress, environmental pollution, lack of exercise, low digestive enzymes and not enough flora (good bacteria) in both the small and large intestine also add to the mucus buildup along the large intestine or colon. Eventually, pockets form along the wall where parasites can populate. As these factors increase, so will heartburn, gas, bloating, ulcers, nausea, constipation, diarrhea, cramps, gas, foul odor and intestinal pain.

Inflammation such as Colitis and diverticulitis occurs. These microforms can actually bore through the colon wall into the blood stream. This allows them to carry the toxins and invade cells, tissues and organs. This stresses the immune system and the liver. As well, our joints contain clear slippery mucus for lubrication. Too much toxic mucus buildup in the body can end up depositing in the joints which contributes to joint stiffness and joint issues.[39] I have personally seen improved joint mobility in clients who went through my cleansing program. Some even reported their chiropractors found their adjustments easier and smoother.

UNHEALTHY CANOLA OIL

One of the hidden health-damaging ingredients added to many foods is canola, a genetically modified, partially hydrogenated oil. It comes from the rapeseed plant, part of the mustard family. Basically, it is an industrial oil, cheap to make, and has been used in candles, soaps, lipsticks, lubricants, inks and bio-fuels. It is not a food. Because of its hybridized and modified state, it can cause health issues. Go with healthier oils like coconut oil, olive oil, organic pastured butter and red palm oil.[40]

BENEFITS OF A RAW VEGETABLE AND FRUIT JUICING CLEANSE

Doing a raw vegetable, fruit juice cleanse is a great way to get rid of the excess mucus build-up along the intestine walls and activate better digestion of your intestinal system.

Cleansing has a huge benefit to bringing the body back to balance. Balance means bringing the body back to where the absorption of nutrients is optimal and there is less inflammation and stress in the body and hormones like insulin, cortisol, and estrogen stay balanced allowing the body to also shed excess weight. Keeping cortisol and estrogen levels in check also affects and keep the thyroid functioning, without it becoming underactive or overactive.[41] There will also be less bloating and better absorption of foods because of the increased enzymes in the raw foods and juices. A healthy bacterial balance in the intestine will be restored with the help at least one capsule of a probiotic supplement in the morning. The system will become more alkaline from an increase in foods such as carrots, beets, celery, etc. The body will get more of all the essential vitamins, minerals, elements, enzymes and proteins to rebuild cells. This allows damaged cells of the body to be healed and the damaged areas of the intestinal wall to also heal. Our bodies will have the energy to carry out their functional, living activities within the organs with ease and we will have greater stamina, alertness and vigour.

One of the main reasons I start people with a cleanse program is to decrease inflammation and minimize allergic reactions to foods such as grains containing gluten, corn, dairy products (especially the non-organic, pasteurized dairy products like cheese, yogurt, milk, etc.), peanuts, alcohol, caffeine and refined sugars and artificial sweeteners. The following foods can be used during the juice cleansing meal program; non-starchy vegetables, all kinds of seeds, all fruits – except oranges, tangerines and grapefruit because they are acidic and if you already are too acidic that may induce inflammation in your system. Eating fruits helps with cleansing because all fruits are about 80 to 90 percent water, plus they have fibre, minerals, vitamins, amino acids and fatty acids that the body needs.[42] Also you should keep the nuts and seeds to about one handful size which is around two ounces per day since they are high in fat. Also, wild fish not from fish farms, free-range eggs and organic skinless chicken are allowed. Stay away from seafood, like shrimps, clams, and oysters, because they feed at the bottom of the ocean and tend to carry more toxins in their meat. Stick to clean forms of protein. Have one serving of fermented soya foods like Tempeh, Miso and Natto. They are high in Vitamin K2 which provides a lot of health benefits like Vitamin D. However, stay away from non-fermented soya foods because here in North America about 90 percent are genetically modified, and the affects shown in lab research is alarming.[43] Visit Dr. Mercola's website and join as a subscriber to his articles on soya.

You will be alarmed at the research results of what GMO soya does. Only use cold-pressed oils like organic olive oil, hemp oil, and sesame oil and use only a tablespoon at a time on your salads and no butter. Keep the fats low, so the liver does not have to work hard and a more efficient cleanse can occur.

HERE ARE SOME OF THE POSITIVE RESULTS THAT OCCUR FROM DOING A CLEANSE:[44]

- Less toxic buildup
- Increased energy
- Improved sleep
- Significant decrease in bloating, acid reflux and indigestion
- Greater control of appetite
- Acute awareness of when the body is truly hungry
- Fewer cravings
- More complete elimination
- Improved digestion, absorption and elimination
- Greater mental clarity, sharpness, memory, alertness and concentration
- Better mental and emotional well-being
- Feeling renewed
- Less addiction to total freedom from addiction to sugars, salts, refined carbohydrates, alcohol, junk foods, caffeine, nicotine
- Weight loss
- Balancing of hormone levels of Insulin, Cortisol and Estrogen
- Thyroid functioning at optimal level
- Cleaner blood, healthier skin
- Reduced allergy symptoms
- Clearer sinuses
- Less mucous in the body

MICRONUTRIENTS AND PHYTOCHEMICALS

You will get concentrated amounts of micronutrients in the fresh raw vegetables and fruit juice. Raw organic vegetables have high amounts of phytochemicals which are super-nutrients that do a lot of work in our bodies to keep it at its healthiest. They help to detoxify cancer-causing compounds, deactivate free radicals, protect against radiation damage, and enable DNA repair mechanisms. When you don't get enough foods that contain these phytochemicals, your body ages faster and is more susceptible to cancer and heart disease.

Foods that contain the most known nutrients are also the ones that contain the most phytochemicals. For optimal health, Dr. Furhman has researched and been taking his clients through his successful high raw foods nutritional programs for the past 20 years. Many of the participants not only lost hundreds of pounds of excess weight but were also healed from high cholesterol, and heart and other chronic diseases. He devised an equation to represent the concept of eating foods that are high in micronutrients per calorie. In other words, you want to eat the foods that have the highest density of micronutrients per amount of calories of that food.

Dr. Fuhrman's Health Equation:
H = N/C
Health = Nutrients/Calories

Your future Health (H) will increase as your Nutrient (N) to Calorie (C) ratio increases

A scoring system was put together by Dr. Fuhrman called the Aggregate Nutrient Density Index or ANDI which assigns a variety of foods based on how many nutrients they deliver to your body for each calorie consumed. Each food score is out of a possible 1,000 based on the nutrients per calorie equation. Food labels only list a few nutrients, but these scores are based on 28 important micronutrients plus other phytochemicals.

In addition to determining the ANDI score, an equal-calorie serving of each food was evaluated based on these nutrients: fibre, calcium, iron, magnesium, phosphorus, potassium, zinc, copper, manganese, selenium, Vitamin A, beta carotene, alpha carotene, lycopene, lutein and zeazanthin, Vitamin E, Vitamin C, thiamine, riboflavin, niacin, pantothenic acid, Vitamin B6, folate, Vitamin B12, choline, Vitamin K, phytosterols, glucosinolates, angiogenesis inhibitors, organosulfides, aromatase inhibitors, resistant starch, resveratrol plus ORAC score. ORAC (Oxygen Radical Absorbance Capacity) is a measure of the antioxidant or radical scavenging capacity of a food. For consistency, nutrient quantities were converted from their conventional measurements of (mg, mcg, IU) to a percentage of their Dietary Reference Intake (DRI). For nutrients that have no DRI, goals were established based on available research and current understanding of the benefits of these factors. [45]

Here is a list of the top 20 foods on the ANDI score, from highest to lowest score:

Kale – 1,000
Collard Greens – 1,000
Mustard Greens – 1,000
Watercress – 1,000
Swiss Chard – 895
Bok Choy – 865
Spinach – 707
Arugula – 604
Romaine – 510
Brussels Sprouts – 490
Carrots – 458
Cabbage – 434
Broccoli – 340
Cauliflower – 315
Bell Peppers – 265
Mushrooms – 238
Asparagus – 205
Tomato – 186
Strawberries – 182
Sweet Potato – 181

Cleansing Meal Program Level Two Instructions

(**Note:** Please pay close attention to the serving sizes suggested. You may need to make changes to accommodate your day and how hungry you are depending on your activity level.)

MORNING ROUTINE

Water: First thing in the morning, drink about three to six glasses of filtered, purified water, depending on how dehydrated you are. If you carry a larger body frame and size you may need more water. You may need as many as eight glasses of water. The recommended amount of water you need per day can be calculated by dividing your bodyweight by two which will give you the number of ounces of water you need. Then divide that by eight to get your number of cups per day. Also, carry your water in high quality stainless steel containers or glass; plastic will leach, over time, known toxic chemicals. Even if there are claims that the plastic is safe like the "polycarbonates", I would still urge glass or stainless steel.[46] Furthermore, if you are an athlete and sweat at a high rate, then it's important to drink more water. You will get dehydrated more quickly than the average person who is not training and perspiring as much.

Fresh fruit: After or while you are drinking your glasses of water, eat a bowl of fresh fruit sprinkled with cinnamon. Fruit is a high-water content food which is digested quickly so it does not interfere with the elimination cycle of the body during the morning period which lasts till noon. Cinnamon, as researched by the National Institute of Health, contains "cinnamaldhyde" which fights against bacterial and fungal infections. It was used to treat colds. The institute also concluded that consuming about six grams of cinnamon per day reduces serum glucose, triglyceride, LDL and cholesterol. In addition, it will reduce total cholesterol in type 2 diabetics.[47] Make sure you wait at least 30 minutes to let the body digest the fruit before you eat your breakfast meal.

Breakfast will be light, high-water content fruits because the body follows three different eight-hour cycles. The morning is when the body goes through its elimination cycle. Therefore, you don't want to consume a lot of solid food that will interfere with this process. This is known as the circadian rhythms.[48]

THE THREE CYCLES ARE:

- Elimination (of body wastes and food debris) 4am-12pm
- Appropriation (eating and digesting) 12pm-8pm
- Assimilation (absorption and use) 8pm-4am

This program is a mixture of clean whole foods, mainly raw vegetable juices and fruits. Hence it is a semi-fast program where you will be replacing some parts of your meals and snacks with a liquid juice; green smoothies and sometimes a vegetarian protein shake. Normally, most of the body's energy is going towards digestion and keeping all the organs of the body functioning. Hence, the body rarely has extra energy to work on itself for repair and cleansing. When we cut down on eating heavy foods that take a lot of digestive energy and consume more liquid juice which takes a lot less energy, the body actually has more extra energy left to work on itself and do needed cleansing. Twenty to 30 percent of the total calories in protein go to digestion. Five to 10 percent of the calories in carbohydrates go to digestion and 0 to three percent of the calories of fat go to digestion. [49] I have developed this Cleansing Meal Program Level Two so you can still eat some solid foods, like salads, fruits and some fish protein, when needed. The other half of the meals will be in the form of fresh juices made from a juicing machine, protein shakes and smoothies. You really won't be hungry. It is a partial fast meal program. Most people can follow this kind of a cleanse and still function in their daily tasks at work and even keep up with training at the gym. However, the training may have to be reduced to a lighter, less intense routine during this period, especially for those who are doing heavy weight training, power-lifting, heavy training on a football team or on a competitive sports team. If you are playing in a sport like hockey or soccer where you burn a lot of calories, you may have to take it easy just for the week you are doing this cleansing program.

MORNING CLEANSING BREAKFAST

Since your body is still in the elimination phase in the morning, it's best not to eat any solid food with the water except some fruit. Fruit is so easily digested, it does not interfere much with the cycle. You wait about 30 minutes and then have about four to eight ounces of a seed cereal. The recipe is shown on the following page. This is basically a raw-food recipe and is a protein cereal which is quite filling and easily digested, so it doesn't disrupt the body's cleansing process. You can add about six ounces of unsweetened almond milk and a teaspoon of pure maple syrup. Breakfast is going to be mainly this seed cereal with vegetable and fruit juices made fresh from a juicer. The vegetable juice can be an eight- to 12-ounce glass depending on how much you can handle. If for some reason you do not have time to make the seed cereal, then you can consume at least an ounce or two of raw almonds or walnuts to get your protein. As much as possible, I suggest you make the seed cereal because it is not only nutritious, but also filling. Seeds are a protein food, so this is a protein cereal. You can make double the serving in the recipe and have it as another small meal later on in the day. I also add a teaspoon of any green powders like Spirulina, Chlorella or Greens Plus to my juice and make it even more potent in nutrients. This is a high enzyme drink which the body will assimilate much faster since it is in liquid form. Hence, it is a micro-nutrient food which the cells of your body will be able to breakdown and absorb more readily than the solid form of the vegetables and fruits.

Vitamins and supplements: This is also the time to take your vitamins and supplements. The benefits of vitamins and supplements will be presented in more detail in the supplement section of this book. It is better to take fat-soluble vitamins with food since some of the fat in the food will help store the vitamin. However, water-soluble vitamins like B and C can be taken in between meals with a glass of water. Sometimes, people can get an upset stomach from taking vitamins on an empty stomach, so to make it gentler I suggest taking them with food. Vitamin C powder should be taken in the morning to help keep your immune system high. I suggest the powder form because it has higher absorption in most brands; almost 25 percent.[50] A minimum of 2,000 mg a day of Vitamin C is essential for our bodies because this is a major anti-oxidant that can help fight off free radicals in the body, kill off viruses and increase the immune system. On days when I feel run down and feel a possible cold coming on, I will double the dose to 2,000 three times during the day with meals. A heaping teaspoon is around 2,000 mg and can be taken with a couple of ounces of water with your meal at breakfast time and supper. The second water-soluble vitamin that everyone needs to take is a B-complex in powder form in a capsule which also has around 25 percent absorption. I recommend a minimum 50 mg capsule of B-complex. Then comes Omega-3. I take three capsules of liquid Omega-3 fish oil from wild salmon or I get it in liquid form in a bottle at the local health food store. You may choose to take this in capsule form as fish oil does not keep long in the fridge and is usually good only for a few months. Also, many people find the taste unappealing.

MID-MORNING

By late morning, around 10:30am or 11:00am, you may be hungry since your breakfast is rather light compared to your usual breakfast meals. If you are not

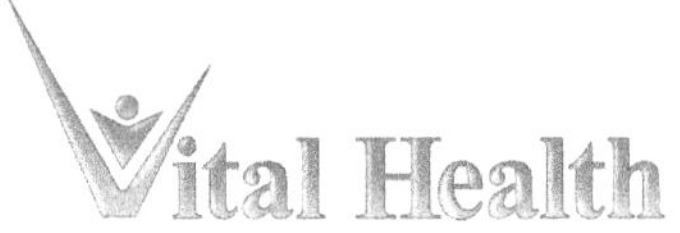

hungry, then just have a cup of herbal tea with maybe a teaspoon of honey. If you are hungry, then eight- to 12-ounces of a Mediterranean shake called Pure Trim is recommended during this cleanse. This is a vegetarian shake mix made from organic peas, brown rice protein, fermented vegetables, nuts, seeds, omega oils, etc. It is very filling, tastes great and highly nutritious. Because it's in liquid form, you won't disrupt the body's cleansing process too much. Drink a glass of water after the shake. This will ensure you are drinking enough water with your food and also helps activate the enzymes of the raw food ingredients in the shake.

LUNCH CLEANSE MEAL

At this time, you will have your second glass of vegetable juice and some solid foods. You don't want to slow down the cleansing process, so consume foods that will not take much digestive energy, like raw vegetables. Different kinds of salads are recommended. For the dressing, use the following ingredients: olive oil (cold-pressed only), freshly squeezed lemon juice, and herbs and seasonings of your choice, like oregano, parsley, cilantro, black pepper and sea salt. For protein, I suggest about four to six ounces of baked or barbequed salmon, or other fish like cod, red snapper, white tuna, etc. Firm tofu is a good alternative protein to have with your salad. The reason for consuming raw vegetables during this period is to infuse the body with as many micro-nutrients as possible. It's the phytochemicals in these raw foods that fight disease and increase your immune system.

If you are heavily into training at the gym or involved in a sport of some kind where you expend a lot of energy, then you may want to take an extra protein shake using the Pure Trim recipe in the instruction section of the book. You can use half a package of Pure Trim to make a two-and-a-half cup of Blender shake or use a whole package if you really need more calories during lunch to fuel your activity level. As shown in the protein shake recipe, you may want to add a banana, six ounces of fruit with the two-and-a-half cups of water and even a few ounces of non-flavoured soya or almond milk to give it a more creamy taste.

I found I needed to consume this amount of protein shakes to sustain my energy for training with weights, floor exercises and cardio. If you are not as active, then you may be fine with just juice and a salad with some fish. I recommend fish because it takes less digestive energy. It is recommended you avoid meats during this time. You can have chicken if you really do not like fish. Remember, this is just a temporary cleanse plan which lasts about a week or two. You will be able to return to a normal level of calorie intake afterwards to keep up with your training.

MID-NOON SNACK

At this time, take your third glass of vegetable juice. If you are still hungry, then take a second Pure Trim shake. If that is still not enough, grab about one ounce of almonds, pecans or walnuts.

SUPPER CLEANSE MEAL

Supper will be very similar to your lunch except you can have some steamed non-starchy vegetables with your four to six ounces of fish or tofu. Some examples of the vegetables are given in the cleanse daily meal sheet. Salad with the meal is recommended. A bowl of vegetable soup is a good addition if you are very hungry. You can get ready-made organic soups in a box at the grocery store or make your own. A personal favourite of mine is the organic butternut squash or roasted pepper tomato soup that you can buy in ready-made boxes. Also drink your fourth glass of vegetable juice here with another teaspoon of vitamin C powder which you can mix in the juice. If you suffer from any kind of joint pain or arthritis, take another two to three capsules or a tablespoon of omega-3 fish oil with your supper to help with the joint pain.

EVENING SNACK

For an evening snack, another four to eight ounces of fresh fruit with a handful of almonds, walnuts or pecans is recommended. You can also have as many cups of herbal tea as you want. In many cases you can confuse thirst with hunger. When you keep hydrated with lots of water and herbal tea, you will not be as hungry.

THE CLEANSING HERBAL SUPPLEMENT "EXPERIENCE"

To further cleanse your system at a deeper level, there is a Mediterranean herbal supplement called Experience which I use that further cleanses the digestive organs and the intestines. It will continue to cleanse while you eat throughout the year. To do a complete body cleanse, we would have to follow a 40-day cleanse just on juices of raw vegetables and fruit – unrealistic for most people therefore we incorporate this herbal supplement. Therefore, I start people with this cleanse program where you still get to partially cleanse your system, then by taking the herbal supplement, Experience, for about a year and half, it eventually cleans your whole system a bit at a time. As long as your eating is balanced with enough raw vegetables, fruits and minimal processed foods, the cleansing will occur. After the year and a half, you will still need to take at least one capsule of Experience in the evening to maintain a clean state of your system. Obviously, many of us still cheat and have meals at restaurants and dinners at other people's homes, where the food may be less than pure, hence your body is always accumulating some toxins from foods eaten. On occasion, I will have a pasta meal at a friend's place that is made with non-organic meat and white, enriched-flour bread. At these times, I always take Experience in the evening before I go to bed, so it will work at digesting and cleansing my system while I sleep. In the morning, excess fats, cholesterol and toxins can be eliminated. This Mediterranean herbal formula traps excess fats and cholesterol in the digestive system. I've had female clients lose five pounds just taking the product without even following my nutritional program. It was developed by Master Herbalist Aboukhazaal who comes from a family line of herbal tradition predating the Chinese and Ayurvedic herbal practices. Experience contains King Solomon Seed, a very strong antioxidant. The ingredients are given on page 83 for you to look at. I have had hundreds of my clients over the years use this product and I myself have been using it for over 10 years. It has many properties and helps with digestion, flatulence, bloating, breaks down gallstones, traps excess fat and cholesterol. You can go to the retail site at vitalcleanse.puretrim.com where you can buy Experience there. It goes for $39 a bottle and there are 90 capsules in a bottle. Please look at my instruction sheet in the next few pages to see how to take it. You can either just swallow the capsule with a glass of water or open the capsule and empty the herbal powder into a mug of warm water and drink it as a tea. You can add half a teaspoon of unpasteurized honey or organic molasses to it which makes it taste nicer or you can take it plain. The molasses makes the tea even more alkaline which is very beneficial to your system, especially if your digestive system is acidic from a meal eaten that had processed food and wrong food combinations. This product may not be for you if you have bleeding ulcers because it may have an irritating effect on the lining of your stomach or intestine which may cause further bleeding. If you have diverticulitis or polyps, you may react to this with diarrhea and frequent bowel movements. There is a normal cleansing reaction of the bowels as they are getting rid of a lot of buildup in the system. Therefore you will have more than normal bouts of eliminations. If you have Crohns, then gently ease into taking a capsule every other day and if the reactions seem normal and your bowel lining is not irritated, then continue. If you have major IBS conditions and are not sure about how your bowels will react, start with one capsule as a tea and if you find you are going to the washroom too much, then take it every other day. Please be aware that you cannot give this to children under 12 years of age or to lactating or pregnant females. If you want to give it to your child under 12 years old because they have severe digestive issues like chronic constipation, then I would get the help of a holistic nutritionist or naturopathic doctor to guide you in the process.

OTHER JUICE RECIPES

Since you will be following this regime for a week minimum, you may get tired of using the same juice recipe, so I have provided extra juice recipe sheets. You can go over them and choose other recipes to try in this week-long cleanse program. However, I strongly suggest you take at least two cups of the carrot with beet recipe as given in the first Seed Cereal, Juice recipe sheet. The other two juices of the day can be any one of your choosing from the other juice recipe sheets. The reason for this is the carrots, beets, celery, apple and ginger recipe have all the right properties to allow cleansing to occur in the body and they contain micro-nutrients that really nourish the cells of the body. It is a very potent combination. Furthermore, after you go through this Cleanse Level Two program for a week take the eighth day to eat some complex, starchy carbohydrates like sweet potato, brown rice, corn or squash. You can also have some beef, steaks, roast beef, etc. Another sheet that I have provided for you is a non-toxic food, soaps, cleaners and essential items list. Most of this can be found at a local health food store or even at many of the organic food sections of major grocery store chains such as Loblaw's Superstore. It will be important for you to make better choices in what kind of foods and everyday essentials you use. After you have done the cleanse, you will want to minimize the amount of toxins going back into your body.

There is a Cleanse Grocery List sheet available in this section of the book after the juice recipes sheets in the following pages. Please refer to it to help you summarize all the supplements, products and foods needed for the cleanse program.

Optional Second Week of Stricter Cleanse

If you feel you can handle it, do another week of the cleanse program to allow the body to cleanse more deeply and get rid of more toxins that have been in the body for years. In the second week, you can be stricter in your eating where you eliminate more solid foods and rely more on juices. This will allow for the body to do a deeper cleanse since you are eating less solid foods which means less energy goes to digestion and more can be spent on repair and cleansing of the body. However, it is a little more challenging, so if you are keeping up with a heavy training program or involved in an intense physical sport like hockey, football or track and field then I would not go this strict. If you still want to do this second week of cleanse, then I suggest you lay your sport or training in the gym aside for a week while you are doing this program. If you have eaten a lot of processed food in the past and have quite a bit of excess fat to lose, then I strongly suggest you do this second week. The second week of the more strict cleanse program is given on another daily cleanse sheet provided in the next few pages. Just follow the instructions given. If you find it too hard to follow after you have started the second week, just add in some of the solid foods that I indicated on the first cleanse daily sheet and you should be able to keep going. If you are someone who is trying to lose a fair amount of weight then I would recommend you do this cleanse program for about four weeks where at

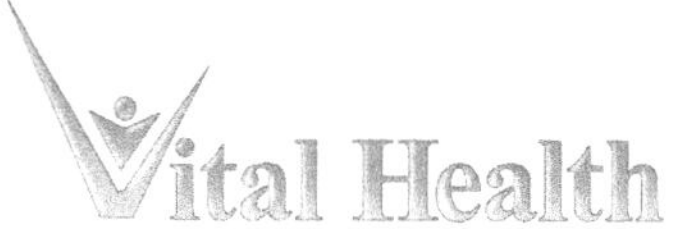

the end of each week of cleanse, have a cheat day on the eighth day by eating some starch like potatoes, brown rice, etc. and some beef, chicken. However, I would stay away from any form of pastas during this cleanse period. They are a processed food and take a lot of energy to digest and are very mucous forming in the intestine. You will find that there will be a significant weight-loss effect from this cleansing program because your liver is being detoxified and will allow for it to break down fat much easier. The reason I suggest people who need to lose a fair amount of fat go through a longer cleansing period, is because excess fat stores a lot of toxins and this is a good way of accelerating the detoxification process and lose some weight faster at the same time. This cleansing program has given a lot of my overweight clients a boost because they come out of this cleanse period leaner and ready to tackle the weight-loss eating program with greater motivation and confidence. The majority of the people come out of this cleanse program with less cravings, slimmer body and a renewed taste for healthier foods. You will have greater energy because of the higher amount of micronutrients in the raw fruit, vegetable juices and raw vegetable salads that you have been eating in the program.

CLEANSING LEVEL TWO DAILY MEAL SHEET

(Appliances needed: Coffee Grinder, Breville Juicer or Samson Extruder and Blender)

(Note: foods in brackets are optional, more juices, shakes, and less solid food results in greater cleanse)

Foods Eaten:

- Minimum 8-10 glasses of filtered or spring water throughout the day or your calculated amount of water according to your body weight.
- Take 1 tsp Vitamin C powder, 1 Vitamin B-complex, 50 mg

First thing in Morning

- Upon waking, drink about 3 - 6 cups of filtered water to rehydrate your body.
- 4-8 oz fruit (i.e. apple, kiwi, melons, strawberry, nectarine and berries are low sugar fruits, consume low sugar fruits if more weight loss is desired from the cleanse)

Breakfast

- 2 - 4 oz seed cereal or 1-2 oz raw almonds
- 8 - 12 oz veg. / fruit juice (one tall glass)
- 1 tbsp Omega-3 fish oil or 3 capsules of the fish oil
- 8 oz Herbal Tea (any herbal tea with 1 tsp honey if desired)

10 a.m. snack:

- 8 -12 oz protein meal replacement shake

Lunch

- 8 oz salad, cold-pressed olive oil, squeezed lemon and 4-6 oz fish, egg or tofu
- 8 - 12 oz veg. / fruit juice (Note: If still hungry, 1 tbsp organic almond butter or 1-2 oz. almonds, cashews)

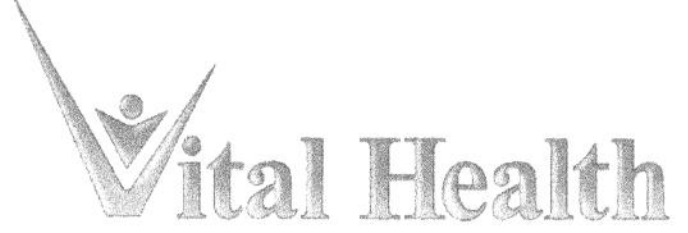

3 p.m. snack:

- 8 - 12 oz protein shake (Note: If still hungry 4-8 oz of fruit and 1-2 oz almonds, pecans or walnuts)
- 8 - 12 oz veg. / fruit juice

Supper

- Take 2nd 1 tsp of Vitamin C powder
- 1 tbsp Omega-3 oil or 3 soft gel capsule form
- 8 - 12 oz veg. / fruit juice
- 4 - 6 oz tuna, fish, chicken or turkey
- 12 oz or more of non-starchy vegetables such as steamed broccoli, carrots, spinach, green beans, kale, spinach, Swiss chard etc.
- 12 oz or more of salad with tbsp olive oil, fresh lemon juice, and herbs and seasonings

Evening Snack

- 4 - 8 oz fruit and/or (handful of almonds, walnuts or pecans)
- 8 oz Herbal Tea (any herbal tea with 1 tsp honey if desired)
- Take 1 - 2 capsules of the Cleansing Herbal supplement Experience

(Note: two servings of juice need to be the carrot recipe; other two can be from the juice recipe sheets)

STRICT CLEANSING LEVEL TWO DAILY MEAL SHEET

(Appliances needed: Coffee Grinder, Breville Juicer or Samson Extruder and Blender)

(Note: foods in brackets are optional, more juices, shakes, and less solid food results in greater cleanse)

Foods Eaten:

- Minimum 8 - 10 glasses of filtered or spring water throughout the day or your calculated amount of water according to your body weight,
- Take 1 tsp Vitamin C powder, 1 Vitamin B-complex, 50 mg

First thing in Morning

- Upon waking, drink about 3 - 6 cups of filtered water to rehydrate your body
- 4 - 8 oz fruit (i.e. apple, kiwi, melons, strawberry, nectarine, etc., 4oz = ½ a cup, consume low sugar fruits if more weight loss is desired from the cleanse)

Breakfast

- 4 - 8 oz seed cereal
- 8 - 12 oz veg. / fruit juice (one tall glass)
- 1 tbsp Omega-3 fish oil or 3 capsules of fish oil
- 8 oz Herbal Tea (any herbal tea with 1 tsp honey if desired)

10 a.m. snack:

- 8 - 12 oz Protein meal replacement shake

Lunch

- (12 oz or more salad, cold pressed olive oil, squeezed lemon and spices)
- 8 - 12 oz veg. / fruit juice
- 3 p.m. snack:
- 8 - 12 oz Protein shake (Note. If hungry 4-8 oz of fruit)
- 8 - 12 oz veg. / fruit juice

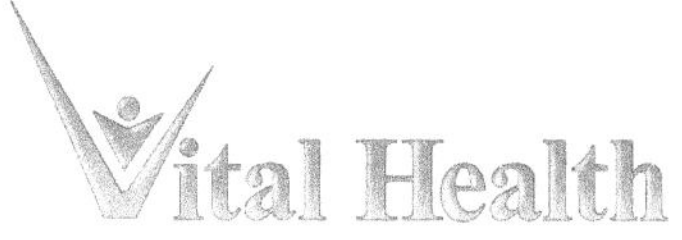

Supper

- Take 2nd 1 tsp of Vitamin C powder
- 1 tbsp Omega-3 oil or 3 soft gel capsule of fish oil
- 8 - 12 oz veg. / fruit juice
- 12 oz or more of salad with tbsp olive oil and fresh lemon juice, spices with 8 oz tofu, 3 oz of almonds, walnuts, pecans or 4-8 oz seed cereal

Evening Snack

- 4 - 8 oz fruit
- 8 oz Herbal Tea (any herbal tea with 1 tsp honey if desired)
- 8 - 12 oz veg. / fruit juice
- Take 1 - 2 capsules of the Cleansing Herbal supplement Experience

(Note. two servings of juice need to be the vegetable/fruit recipe; other ones can be your choice from the juice recipe sheets)

SEED, JUICE, & PROTEIN SHAKE RECIPES

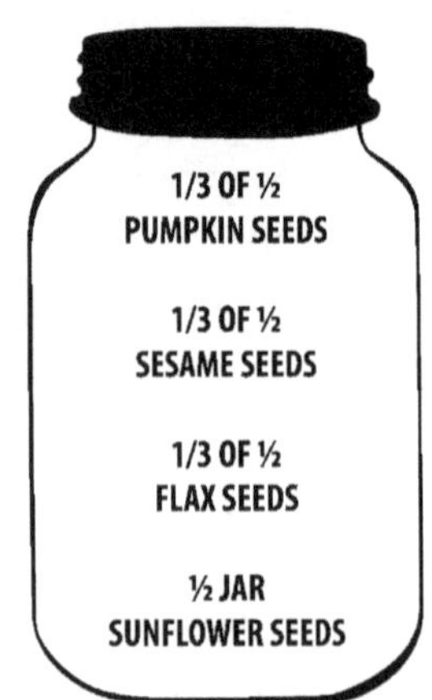

Single Serving Seed Cereal Recipe

(Approx. 4 - 5 oz serving; use coffee grinder)

- 1 heaping tbsp Sesame seeds (raw seeds)
- 1 heaping tbsp Flax seeds (with skin on)
- 3 - 4 heaping tbsp Sunflower seeds (raw hulled)
- 1 heaping tbsp Pumpkin seeds (raw hulled)

Fill half of an empty large pickle or mason glass jar with the sunflower seeds. Then fill the other top half of the jar with a 1/3 pumpkin seeds, 1/3 Flax seeds and 1/3 Sesame seeds. It does not have to be exact. You will have approximately the same ratio of seed mixture as prescribed for the single serving recipe given. Then you can just scoop out 5-6 heaping tbsp of the mixture into the coffee grinder and grind to the desired consistency. Then empty into a bowl, add your boiled water by trickling it in slowly until its texture becomes like a porridge. You can also sprinkle some crushed cashews, walnuts, and a teaspoon of unpasteurized honey or maple syrup. Finally add about 4 - 8 ounces of goat's milk, rice milk or unsweetened almond milk and you are ready to eat. Store seeds in a glass jar. Mix well and keep in the fridge to keep seeds fresher or in a cool dry place.

Four Cup Juice Recipe

- 9 - 10 medium size carrots (source of High Beta-carotene)
- 2 celery sticks (source of Sodium)
- 1 - 2 apples (Macintosh, Empire or Spartan, source of Vitamin C)
- 1 or ½ medium size beet (Natural Blood Cleanser, source of Iron)
- 2-inch chunk fresh ginger root (Anti-viral, Anti-bacterial)

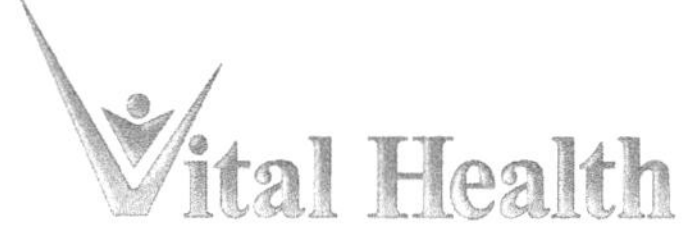

Three Cup Protein Shake Recipe
(Use glass blender if possible, easier to clean)

- ½ banana or 1 whole banana
- 1 or ½ pack of Pure Trim (Note: for additional protein add one or two 30 g. scoop of non-flavoured whey isolate protein powder if you need more protein, especially if you are training a lot in the gym and doing intense aerobic activity)
- 2 ½ cups of water
- 4 - 6 oz of strawberries, blueberries, pineapples or fruit of your choice
- 2 oz of unsweetened almond milk or goat's milk (Optional)

JUICE RECIPES

IRON SUPPORT	
3 beet tops, 1 beet, handful of parsley, handful of organic spinach, 4 - 5 carrots, 2 organic kale leaves	Bunch up kale, parsley, spinach, beet tops, and beet then push through the hopper with carrots
CUCUMBER MIX FOR SKIN (ECZEMA)	
1 tomato, handful of organic spinach, 1 carrot, 1 cucumber, 2 organic celery stalks, parsley for garnish	Juice tomato, spinach, cucumber, carrot, and celery, then pour juice into tall glass; garnish with sprig of parsley
MELON SHAKE FOR BLADDER	
1 cantaloupe with green part of skin, 2 - 3 carrots, 1 - 2 organic apples	Peel cantaloupe's outer skin, cut in strips and put through hopper with carrots and apples
BRONCHITIS SPECIAL	
1 pineapple with green skin, 1 cucumber, 2-3 kiwi	Push pineapple through hopper with cucumber and kiwi
JOINT REMEDY	
1 large bunch of grapes 2 organic apples (seeded), ½ cantaloupe, 1 lemon wedge	Push grapes and cantaloupe through hopper with apples and lemon
BURSITIS CITRUS	
2 - 3 oranges, 1 lemon (peeled), 1 ½ organic apple (seeded)	Push oranges, lemon, and apples through hopper
CARPAL TONIC	
¼ pineapple with skin, ½ organic apple (seeded), kiwi, organic celery, ¼ inch slice ginger root	Push pineapple through hopper with apple, kiwi, celery, and ginger
CUT CHOLESTEROL SHAKE	
½ orange (peeled & leave white part), ½ papaya (peeled), 1 banana, 1 carrot, 3 organic strawberries, Orange twist for garnish	Push orange, carrot, and strawberries through hopper with papaya, then place juice and banana in blender or food processor and blend until smooth

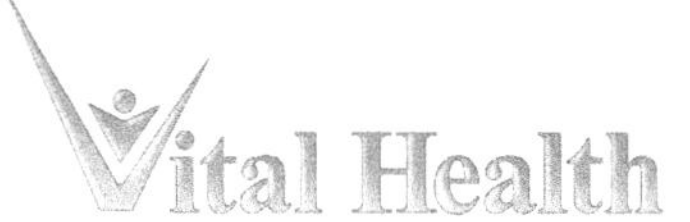

ADDITIONAL JUICE RECIPE LIST

COOL-DOWN SPLASH	WHEATGRASS ENERGY DRINK
3 Carrots 3 Organic Strawberries 2 Kiwis 3 Cauliflower ¼ Red Cabbage	1 Handful of Wheatgrass 1 Handful of Organic Spinach 1 Pineapple Spear 1 Handful of Swiss Chard
DAILY DETOX	**FRESH PAPAYA JUICE**
6 Stalks Asparagus (Remove Fibrous End) ½ Lemon ½ Organic Cucumber 1-2 Carrots	1 Large Ripe Papaya (Peel and seeds Removed) 1 oz Organic Grapes
DIGESTIVE JUMP START	**WATERMELON JUICE**
½ Papaya (Peeled and seeds removed) 1 Organic Apple 1 Guava (peeled and seeds removed) 2 Spears of Pineapple	½ a Watermelon Remove and Cut Watermelon into pieces that will fit easy into the chute.
SUPER BOOST	**THINK DRINK**
3 Tomatoes ¼ Organic Red Pepper ¼ Green Pepper 2 Cloves of Garlic ¼ Jalapeno (optional) ¼ Onion (Peeled) 1 Organic Celery Stalk 1 Carrots 1 - 2 ½ inch slice of Cabbage Add to juice in listed order*	1 Passion Fruit 1 Organic Apple 1 Piece of Ginseng 1 - 2 oz Almond Milk
LIGHTEN UP	**THROAT COAT**
½ Organic Apple ¼ Cantaloupe (Rind Removed) 6 Edges of Watermelon (Rind Removed) ½ Grapefruit 2-3 Kiwis	Handful of Wheat Grass Wrapped in Organic Kale or Swiss Chard 1 Unpeeled Lemon 3 Pineapple Spears

CANTALOUPE CALMER	SKIN GLOW
½ Cantaloupe (Rind Removed) 2 Pears Add coconut for an exotic treat*	1 Organic Cucumber ½ Cup of Organic Parsley 1 Apple 4 Carrots Add ¼ - ½ cup Coconut Milk or Almond milk
CARROT FRUIT JUICE	**FRESH PINEAPPLE & CARROT JUICE**
4 Large Carrots 2 Sweet organic apples, such as red or golden delicious	4 Large Carrots ½ Pineapple (cut into spears)[51]

Pure Trim Products Instructions

EXPERIENCE

100% natural digestive support formula for cleansing the bowels, removing fat and promoting regularity.

Most effective as a tea: Empty 1 or 2 capsules into a cup of pre-heated warm water; 2 teaspoons of Harmony or ½ teaspoon of molasses or honey may be added

> Start with one capsule daily for the first 3 days at bedtime or 30-60 minutes after a meal, if stomach is sensitive.
>
> Increase to 2 capsules if you find 1 is not enough until you achieve desired results, such as more frequent bowel movements, some mild cleansing reactions in the body, such as mild diarrhea and watery stool. Also, the odd pimple may appear since the body may be getting rid of toxins through the skin.
>
> The amount required may vary depending on size of person and bowel condition, and level of toxic buildup in the body, etc. Therefore, be observant of your results; 2 - 4 capsules per day are usually sufficient.

Do not take Experience at the same time as medication; take it 3 - 4 hours apart from time of taking medication.

Avoid or reduce intake of salt, carbonated beverages and caffeine for best results

Drink 8 - 10 glasses of water minimum per day for best results.

Take 1 capsule of Experience daily for the first week, then 2 capsules daily for the next 12 months and 1 - 2 capsules daily as maintenance after that.

HARMONY

Natural food for balancing body chemistry's strengthening your immune system, increasing energy and for overall well-being. Also helps with acid reflux issues.

Take 1 - 2 teaspoons, 1 - 2 times daily. For best results, take on an empty stomach by itself, in cold water or in warm water as a tea. If taking as a tea, use warm water before adding Harmony.

You may use Harmony with Experience.

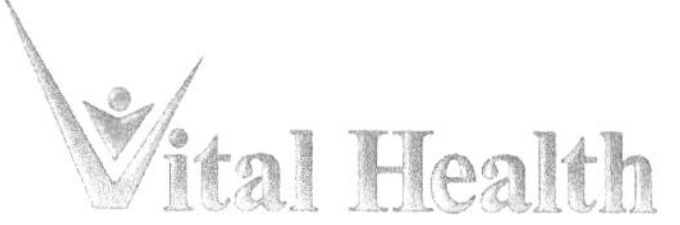

PURE TRIM SHAKE RECIPE

(Use glass blender if possible, easier to clean)

½ a banana or 1 whole banana (drink a glass of water after)

Half a package of Pure Trim

2 ½ cups of water

2 oz of unsweetened almond milk or goat's milk

(Optional: 4 - 6 oz of strawberries, blueberries or a fruit of your choice)

SYNERGY PRO-BIOTIC CAPSULES

Take 1 capsule with a glass of water before or during largest meal of the day. This adds more good bacteria in the intestine so it will aid digestion and help absorb food better. This also helps increase the immune system.

DAILY COMPLETE

Take 1 or half an ounce during or after a meal. Shake well before use. You can also mix with other organic unpasteurized juices or water to dilute it if you don't like it thick. Always drink a glass of water after. Refrigerate after opening.

CLEANSING PROGRAM GROCERY LIST

Products:

- Experience (cleansing product available at: vitalcleanse.puretrim.com)
- Vitamin C (powder or capsules: available at local health food stores)
- Vitamin B Complex (50-100mg capsules, available at local health food stores)
- Pure-Trim Shake (vanilla, strawberry or chocolate, available at: vitalcleanse.puretrim.com)
- Synergy (probiotic available at: vitalcleanse.puretrim.com)
- Omega-3 Fish Oil Soft Gel (capsules or liquid, available at health food stores
- Harmony (available at: vitalcleanse.puretrim.com)
- Daily Complete (available at: vitalcleanse.puretrim.com)

Seed Mixture & Nuts (available at local health food stores)

- Sunflower seeds (raw, hulled)
- Flax seeds (raw)
- Dark sesame seeds (raw with skin)
- Pumpkin Seeds (raw, no skin)
- Unsalted roasted or raw almonds
- Organic Molasses

Produce for Juicing (available at local health food stores)

- Carrots
- Celery
- Loose Beets or with the leaves on
- Apples (Mac, Empire, Spartan etc)
- Ginger Root
- Kale

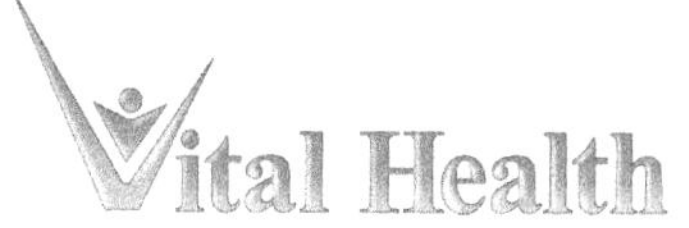

EXPERIENCE INGREDIENTS

Psyllium Seed Husk (Plantaga Orata)
Stimulates Bowel Peristalsis

Senna Leaves (Senna Anguslifalia)
Purgative, stimulates peristalsis; helps with constipation

Fennel Seed (Fremonluim Vulagaire)
Carminative meaning to expel gas from the stomach, intestines, Expectorant, to expel mucus from the respiratory area

Corn Silk (Stigmata Maydis)
Diuretic, edema, prostate disorders, reduces kidney stone formation

Solomon's Seal (Rhizame Polygamative Multiflora)
Astringent, contract tissue, demulcent, soothes inflammation of the bowels, tonic

Kelp (Fuans Vesicaulons)
Rich in iodine/alkali, helps convert indigestible sugars, (i.e. Beans) thus reduce gas, flatulence

Black Seed (Nigella Sativa)
Helps skin, stomach, intestinal disorders, kidney and liver functions, circulatory, immune system (I.S.), vegetable Cellulose [52]

NON-TOXIC FOODS & NATURAL ESSENTIALS

Local Health Food Store:
Organic bread
(Sprouted Ezekiel bread, Manna bread, Spelt, Kamut bread)
Non-pasteurized honey
Pure maple syrup
Sucanat (dehydrated sugar cane juice)
Oatmeal
Millet (gluten free, alkaline grain)
Quinoa
Seeds
Organic kale, Swiss chard, spinach, and romaine
Free range eggs
Raw cheese
Goat's milk
Organic yogurt
Organic apples, blueberries, and strawberries,
Organic peanut butter & almond butter
Agave nectar
Organic molasses
Non-pasteurized juices
Mary's Organic crackers (gluten free) Kasha (organic cracker)
Salad dressing & dip mixes
Inca (coffee substitute drink mix)
Boxed organic soups
Soba noodles (Asian or Korean Food Store)
Chinese vermicelli
Dried vegetable chips
Organic natural potato chips
Vegetarian bacon bits
Organic jam sweetened with grape juice

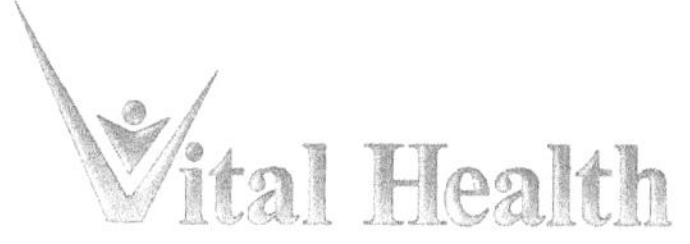

Apple butter (very low calories)
Omega Oils
Prunes, dates, figs (dried with no oil)
(Soak dried fruits in water overnight)
Organic mayonnaise
Thai Kitchen rice noodles
Organic Ramen wheat noodles
Miran (Japanese sauce)
Herbal Teas
Hummus
Chicken & vegetable samosas
Chapati (flat yeast free Indian bread)
Sunflower, Flax, Sesame Seeds
Chicken soup mix (non-msg)
Himalayan sea salt
Cold-pressed olive oil
Organic coffee
Miso Paste
Tempe
Natto
Organic meat, fish

Middle Eastern Food Store:
Babagonush
Tzatziki
Hummus
Dates, Figs
Almonds, Cashews, Walnuts

Local Health Food Store:
Pure Glycerine Soap
Seventh Generation dish soap

Jason shampoo,
Mouth Wash
Jason underarm deodorant
Tee Tree Oil
Uncle Tom's toothpaste
Soap works
Static free drying sheets (Melaleuca.com)
Pure Gardens Cream (vitalcleanse.puretrim.com)
Aura Acacia moisturizing oils
Apricot seed oil
Grape seed oil
Essential oils air freshener
Cream for Dry Skin (beesweetontario.com)
Baked goods from organic grains

Costco Store:
Baby Carrots
Sugar Snaps
Frozen Wild Salmon
Bag of Walnuts
Frozen Fruits
Organic Peas
Almond milk
Mozzarella Cheese
Free Range Whole Chicken

General Parasite Cleanse

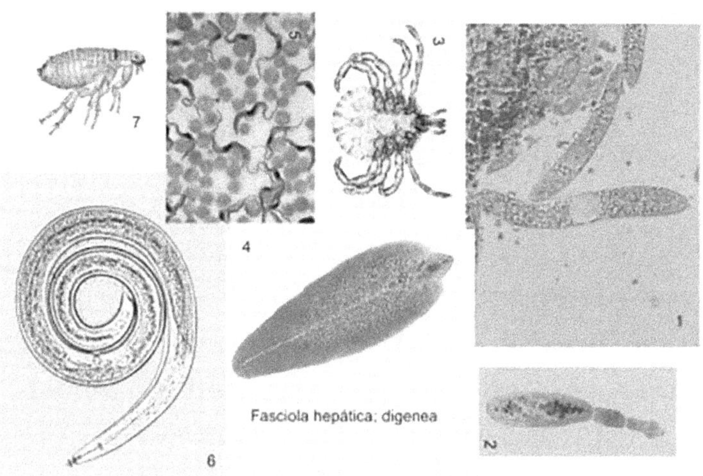

It is a fact that microbial parasites invade human bodies all over the world, in all races. It is estimated that more than 150-million Americans have some kind of parasite feeding in their body. They feed off your vitamins, nutrients and amino acids; making the body more acidic, causing fatigue and compromising health. Therefore, it is crucial for people to watch what foods they eat and use an herbal anti-parasite supplement to combat these invaders. These microforms not only ingest our nutrients, but excrete their own toxins which can affect our immune systems negatively, which then leads to sickness, diseases and other health challenges.

The different ways you can contract them is from handling your pets, kissing your pets, handling animal products, not washing your hands after handling your pet's waste or human waste, walking barefoot, handling dirty objects, human contact, water, eating raw fruits, vegetables, and eating under-cooked meats and fish. One of the huge factors that contribute to this is that many people do not wash their hands after going to the washroom which spreads the contamination of parasites to an enormous level.[53]

The best way to do a general parasite cleanse is by using Clear, a herbal product made by Pure Trim a company that carries some of the products that I use for my cleansing programs. Please go to vitalcleanse.puretrim.com to order.

To eliminate the parasites residing in our body this Spiking program taught by Mediterranean Master Herbalist Aboukhazaal is effective. The evidence of microscopic parasites leaving the body is when you see air bubbles leaving the stool floating to the top of the toilet bowl, or a cloudy-like film on the surface of the toilet bowl. Also, a really unusual smell is also an indication. This program is not for children but adults 18 and over. If you have a child that you want to introduce this to, please take your child to a Naturopath so they can give proper guidance on how to do this type of cleanse. If you have a sensitive body then work your way up to a comfortable amount. Don't take the full dose recommended by this program. For example, if you have taken 3 capsules a day and you move up to 4 capsules a day for a following week, and your body is reacting strongly, then move back to 3 capsules a day for a week, then to 2 capsules for a week, then back to 3 capsules for a week until you finish the three month cycle. Follow the same spiking periods but just take less number of capsules for each week.

WEEK 1	1 capsule with 8 oz water each morning about an hour before breakfast, on an empty stomach.
WEEK 2	2 capsules with 8 oz water each morning one hour before breakfast, on an empty stomach.
WEEK 3	(3 capsules total) 2 capsules with 8 oz water each morning one hour before breakfast on an empty stomach. 1 capsule between lunch and dinner.

WEEK 4	(4 capsules total) 2 capsules with 8 oz water each morning one hour before breakfast, on an empty stomach. 2 capsules between lunch and dinner
WEEK 5	(5 capsules in total) 2 capsules with 8 oz water each morning one hour before breakfast; on an empty stomach. 2 capsules between lunch and dinner. 1 capsule a few hours after supper
WEEK 6	(4 capsules total) 2 capsules with 8 oz water each morning one hour before breakfast, on an empty stomach. 2 capsules between lunch and dinner
WEEK 7	(3 capsules total) 2 capsules with 8 oz water each morning one hour before breakfast on an empty stomach. 1 capsule between lunch and dinner.
WEEK 8	2 capsules with 8 oz water each morning one hour before breakfast on an empty stomach
WEEK 9	1 capsule with 8 oz water each morning each morning one hour before breakfast on an empty stomach
WEEK 10	2 capsules with 8 oz water each morning one hour each morning before breakfast on an empty stomach.
WEEK 11	(3 capsules total) 2 capsules with 8 oz water each morning one hour before breakfast on an empty stomach. 1 capsule between lunch and dinner.
WEEK 12	(4 capsules total) 2 capsules with 8 oz water each morning one hour before breakfast, on an empty stomach. 2 capsules between lunch and dinner

(This program is a 12 week (3 month) program and requires total of 3 family size Clear bottles)

Your diet during the week of the parasite cleanse should consist primarily of:

- Steamed or raw green/non-starchy vegetables.
- Tofu or vegetable protein flakes (TVP) are recommended as meat replacements, but you may eat some fish and chicken (preferably wild or free range).
- Decrease dairy products, to once a week
- Starchy vegetables, such as potatoes, brown rice and yams; consume every 4 days
- Eat one piece of Fruit a day,
- Cut out sugar, honey, molasses, maple syrup or anything else containing sugar, naturally occurring or otherwise.
- Avoid fruit juices

Following the 12 week parasite cleanse, with the left over amount of capsules in the bottle, continue taking 2 Clear™ capsules one hour before breakfast on an empty stomach until the bottle is finished.

(Note: Some fatigue or weakness may be experienced during this cleanse, this is normal and is often the result of lowered blood sugar levels. You may snack on raw vegetables and Tahini dip or Hummus.)

Kidney Cleanse

Since we have gone through the cleansing of our intestines with the juicing program, we need to cleanse the kidneys as well. The kidneys do a tremendous amount of work in the body, controlling and regulating many of the body's functions. One of the main jobs is that they filter and detoxify. They control and have an effect on the various areas of the body like our hearing, gums, teeth, lymphatic system, bones, fertility, energy, strength, balance, lungs, etc.. If they are weak, congested and not functioning at their optimal these are some of the signs that appear in the body. You have loss of hearing, low sex drive, infertility, weak nails, foggy head, low back pain, low energy, bladder issues, poor physical development, swelling and kidney stones.

A kidney cleanse consists of mainly drinking a herbal blend that you can go and buy at the various Health Food stores which sell various herbal mixtures for the cleanse.

You make a tea with the loose herb formula. It dissolves congested residue of salts, minerals, uric acid and proteins in the kidneys. This cleanse usually is for 30 days.

If you have had stones, kidney related health issues, chronic swelling, water retention or chronic illness, this cleanse should be carried out for at least 6 weeks. Then you should repeat one more time during the year for maintenance if you have a diet that is fairly high in meat fats, starches and sugars. If you have a healthy diet that is high in raw fruits, vegetables, whole grains, seeds, nuts and little meat then I would suggest every two to three years do a month of this cleanse.

The kidney tea formula usually is made from the following herbs such as Marjoram, Cat's Claw, Comfrey Root, Fennel Seed, Chicory Herb, Uva Ursi, Hydrangea Root, Gravel Root, Marshmallow Root and Golden Rod.

FOODS TO AVOID AND CONSUME DURING CLEANSE

For best results you need to stay away from red meat, alcohol, table salt, diet foods and drinks, fake sugars. All supplements with synthetic minerals and synthetic vitamin C which is usually ascorbic acid. If you have kidney stones you need to stay away from foods high in oxalic acid like spinach, beets, collard greens, Swiss chard, rhubarb, parsley, okra, peanuts, peanut butter and chocolate. In addition avoid all processed

foods and packaged foods that contain preservatives, sodium, table refined salt, artificial colors and refined sugars. Processed salt is damaging to the kidneys but unrefined sea salt contains minerals and help support the kidneys.

The foods you should eat are beans, vegetables (especially cabbage), non-GMO whole organic grains, fruits, healthy oils, raw nuts and seeds. You can also add fresh vegetable, fruit juice to your diet using some organic vegetables like kale, carrots, celery, water melon, lemons, apples etc.

DIRECTIONS FOR MAKING THE TEA:

In a glass container (not plastic), soak 3 tablespoons of the loose tea in 2 cups of purified water overnight. Do not soak tea in tap water or distilled water. In the morning bring the tea to a low boil for 5 minutes (do not boil on high). Cool and strain. If you forget to soak the tea overnight, boil the tea on low for 15 minutes in the morning. Since some water will boil off, add 3 cups of water instead of 2 cups, and use a lid to prevent the water from evaporating. Drink one cup in the morning about 45 minutes after breakfast and second cup 45 minutes after supper.

* Feel free to add flavor to the tea (it is bitter) such as; flavored tea, lemon juice, raw honey, coconut sugar or agave.

*Do not take with food- wait at least 45 minutes before meals.

Important Note: If you experience discomfort or stiffness in the low back area, do not be alarmed. This indicates that stones are dissolving and mineral crystals are moving through the ureters and urinary tract system. Any strong smell or darkening of the urine also indicates a major release of toxins. It should pass within a few days. Typically, most people experience few or no symptoms. This cleanse is gentle and works gradually over time.

Another way to get the kidney cleanse tea is to order the Kidney Cleanse Kit from this website: **frequencyrising.com.** The one drawback is it takes about 6 weeks or more to receive the shipment from California, USA if you live in the Eastern part of Canada.

Here are the main components in Dr. Clark's Kidney Cleanse, just follow the instructions on the sheet that comes with the products. You have to take the extra supplements along with the tea for kidney support:

KIDNEY SUPPORT TEA 2.5 OZ. BAGS (HYDRANGEA, MARSHMALLOW, GRAVEL ROOTS)
Ginger Root, 500 mg, 63 cts Uva Ursi, 500 mg, 63 ct Vitamin B6, 230 mg, 21 ct Magnesium Oxide, 300 mg, 21 ct Vitamin B2, 230 mg, 21 ct Freeze Dried Parsley 385 mg 42 ct Contains vegetable caps, from Pine Bark Step-by-step instruction sheet

Liver Flush

Once we have cleansed the intestine and the kidneys, we are ready for the next organ to cleanse; the liver and gallbladder. I have revised the liver flush from a combination of a few different liver flush programs introduced by various health practitioners over the past number of years. You will see them in the bibliography at the end of the book. Remember to keep taking the Experience cleansing supplement in the evenings throughout this flush program. Experience actually breaks down stones.

If you are very toxic, carrying 30Ibs or more in excess weight and have consumed a lot of processed foods over the past number of years, then I would recommend you take an extra liver supplement called the Liver Master which is a herbal blend that you can order on the retail site at: vitalcleanse.puretrim.com. It's easy to follow. You just take one capsule with a glass of water twice a day for 90 days. Each pack contains 30 herbal capsules, so two packs for each month is required. This will further detoxify the liver at a deeper level. However, if you cannot afford to, then just do this flush every two weeks until you pass all the stones out of your body. Usually you will need to do this flush at least three times in a row to pass most of the stones. Here are the main things you need to buy for this program:

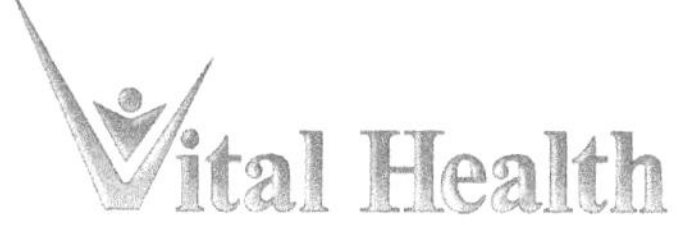

SHOPPING LIST

- Organic unsweetened Cranberry Juice (1 Litre)
- Internal Epsom Salts (4 Tablespoons)
- Cold-Pressed, Light, Organic Olive Oil (½ Cup)
- Fresh pink grapefruit (1 Large or 2 Small - enough to squeeze - ¾ cup or more)
- Organic Apple Cider Vinegar (7 Tablespoons)
- ½ to ¾ cup of unpasteurized honey or pure maple syrup

It's best to schedule the sixth and seventh day of the flush on a weekend. You start on a Friday and finish the program on a Saturday morning then flushing out the stones in the afternoon. This will give you time to rest and recover by the evening so your system will be back to normal by Monday and you can return to normal functioning.

DAY ONE

Drink the amount of water according to your bodyweight which is your weight divided by two which gives a total in ounces, divide by eight to get your number of cups. Four ounces every hour to ensure you are properly hydrated is a good habit. Timing is CRITICAL for success. Please do not be more than 10 minutes early or late in regards to the steps pertaining to taking the apple cider vinegar, Epson salt drink and the olive oil, grapefruit mixture. You will be taking the organic apple cider vinegar every two hours. This softens the stones so they flush out easily without causing pain.

7:00 am to 7:30 am: Eat a non-fat breakfast of some fruit, oatmeal or seed mixture cereal, vegetable juice and a green smoothie of your choice. An additional vegetarian protein shake (Pure Trim shake) will also give you the adequate amount of nutrients, calories and protein you need. A piece of organic whole grain toast with a tablespoon of organic naturally sweetened jam is another good choice to have with the cereal and fruit. (no fat, no processed foods of any kind, no meat, no nuts, no refined sugared foods)

12:00 pm: Eat a non-fat lunch. For example you can have a plate of steamed vegetables, half a sweet potato or squash with some baked firm tofu seasoned with a teaspoon of tamari sauce and sesame seeds. As a healthy side dish, a tossed green garden salad of your choice and fresh lemon juice dressing with some fresh parsley, cilantro, garlic, sea salt, oregano and fresh ground black pepper will help to make it a more filling and tasty meal. I strongly suggest you have a sufficient breakfast and lunch so you can sustain the semi-fast period from 2pm till bedtime.

2:00 pm: Take one tablespoon of apple cider vinegar and chase it down with some water if desired. DO NOT EAT OR DRINK ANYTHING OTHER THAN WATER AFTER 2 pm. If you break this rule, you may feel ill later.

Prepare Epsom Salt solution: Mix 4 tablespoons of Epsom salts with 4 cups unsweetened cranberry juice. Add about ½ cup to ¾ cup of unpasteurized honey or pure maple syrup to sweeten the sourness because it is extremely tart. The Epsom Salt helps clear stagnant waste by activating bowel movements. It also helps dilate the bile ducts of the liver. This makes 4 servings of 1 cup each.

4:00 pm: Take the second tablespoon of apple cider vinegar and chase it down with water again if needed.

6:00 pm: Drink first serving (1 cup) of Cranberry juice Epsom Salt mixture. (Stir before serving to ensure salts are dissolved), in addition, take your third tablespoon of apple cider vinegar.

8:00 pm: Drink your second serving (1 cup) of Cranberry juice / Epsom Salt mixture and take your fourth tablespoon of apple cider vinegar. Get ready for bed and get all chores done.

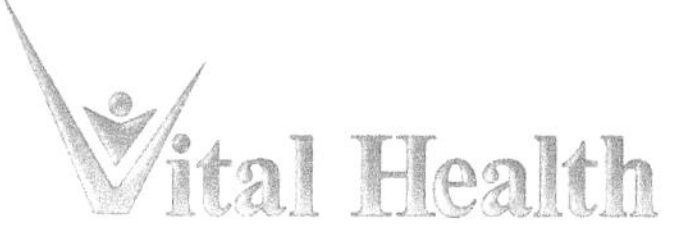

9:30 pm: Prepare olive oil: pour ½ cup olive oil into a glass mason jar. Prepare the squeezed grapefruit juice and measure out 3/4 cup. Add this to the half cup of olive oil. Close the jar tightly and shake hard until watery (only fresh grapefruit should be used). Do not prepare too early as you want fresh enzymes of the grapefruit. Visit the washroom one or more times.

10:00 pm: Drink the olive oil mixture, but drink it standing up. Get it down within 5 minutes. Drinking through a large plastic straw may help this go down easier. Take your fifth tablespoon of apple cider vinegar.

10:10 pm: Make sure you are completely ready for bed ahead of time. As soon as the drink is down, walk to your bed and lie down flat on your back with your head high up on the pillow. This is all part of the body positioning to allow the stones to travel out of the liver ducts. Try to visualize what is happening in the liver. Try to keep perfectly STILL FOR AT LEAST 20 MINUTES. You may feel a train of stones travelling along the bile ducts like marbles. There is no pain because the bile ducts have been opened by the Epsom salts.

AFTER lying still for 20 minutes, go to sleep for the night. Make sure you have set your alarm for 6:00 am. You can get up to go to the washroom after this time if you need to, but not before!

DAY TWO

6:00 am: As soon as you wake up, take your third serving (1 cup) of Cranberry juice Epsom Salt mixture. If you have indigestion or nausea, wait until it is gone before drinking the Epsom salts, but don't take it before 6:00 am. Take the sixth tablespoon of apple cider vinegar. If you wish, you may go back to bed and set your alarm for 8:00 am.

8:00 am: Take your fourth and final serving (1 cup) of Cranberry juice Epsom salt mixture. Take your final seventh tablespoon of apple cider vinegar.

Usually around this time, you will have urges to eliminate. You may have to go every 30 minutes or so. I went about 5 to 6 times on my first flush, so stay close to the washroom. I would not have guests or be doing anything involved. Stay focused on this whole experience of cleansing. You are preventing yourself from any potential future health issues of gallbladder attacks and possibly even unnecessary surgery. It will be mostly liquid with some bile which may be dark greenish in colour with stones. If you are curious, you can use a straightened coat hanger wire and swish it around and you should see some stones floating in your toilet bowl!

10:00 am: Take some fresh fruit juice, preferably prepared fresh in a juicer.

10:30 am: Eat high-water content fruit (i.e. melons, peaches, kiwi, nectarines, etc.)

11:30 am: Eat light, easy-to-digest food; a light NO-FAT breakfast, as shown earlier, and a no-fat light lunch which will allow you to pass more stones – probably later. Stick to vegetables, fruit, oatmeal and herbal tea. Stay away from any meats, fats, oils, dairy products or processed food of any kind. You may or may not continue to pass stones throughout the day till about early to late noon, depending on how many stones you may have. You should be recovered by 10:00 pm -11:00 pm. Your body is in a sensitive state during this time. Don't disrupt the cleansing process. If you cheat, you may aggravate it and feel sick. You can have a colon irrigation done to further flush any remaining stagnant waste, gallstones and parasites that can thrive in the toxic buildup and dwell among the stones. I suggest you consult a colon therapist within a week of your flush. Milk thistle is a good supplement to take for the liver after a flush. Take 1 or 2 capsules a day for about two weeks. This helps the liver heal after the flush experience.

Gentle Liver Cleanse

For those of you who are not ready to go through the seven-day flush, I have also provided this less intense liver cleanse program. It takes much longer, but you can still receive the same results. I would recommend you take an extra liver supplement called the Liver Master, which is a herbal blend that you can order at vitalcleanse.puretrim.com. It's easy to follow. You take one capsule with a glass of water twice a day for 90 days. Each pack contains 30 herbal capsules. You will need two packs each month. This will further detoxify the liver at a deeper level while you are going through this gentle liver cleanse period. However, if you cannot afford this, then just do this liver cleanse month on and month off until you pass all the stones out of your body.

CLEANSING RECIPE

- 1 tbsp Olive Oil
- 1 tbsp Apple Cider Vinegar
- 1 tbsp Lemon Juice
- 1 tbsp of Internal Epsom Salt

Put all these ingredients in 8 - 12 oz. of water and take it before bedtime

Take one to two capsule of a probiotic supplement and one capsule of milk thistle after breakfast each day

Take one to two capsules of Experience (Cleansing Herbal formula) in the evening or before bedtime (Mentioned in the previous cleanse section)

Implement this regiment throughly for a month, then a month off, and then a month on until urine is clear. Urine will be cloudy with the passing of broken gallstone crystals. There are no side effects or discomfort. Stones will be broken down and released as fine powdered crystals.

Remember to drink enough water according to your bodyweight. (Your weight divided by 2 which gives a total in ounces, then divided by 8 to get the number of cups.) The water needs to be made alkaline. Do this by adding 1 - 2 tbsp of liquid chlorophyll to the water you will drink throughout the day. You can also add slices of fresh lemon to make it alkaline.

While on this program, stick to a meal plan that avoids saturated or polyunsaturated fat, foods with refined sugars, wheat, or fried foods. All processed foods, foods made with refined flour, sodas and coffee need to be eliminated. Follow the meal plans from this book for lean males and females and you should be fine.

On your month off, you can eat foods such as these:

Fish oil
Cold-pressed olive oil
Natural unpasteurized honey
Maple syrup
Organic grains
Vegetables
Fruits
Organic sprouted bread
Seeds and nuts
Some organic coffee
Herbal teas
Lean organic meat
Poultry
Wild unfarmed fish
Fermented tofu
Miso
Beans
Lentil

Basic Heavy Metal Cleanse

Again, I am not an expert, but I try to eliminate as much as possible the use of everyday products that contain heavy metals. The cleansing programs I have introduced in this book help clear toxins from the body which will include some heavy metals. Products, like Experience, help with this as well, however, heavy metals are everywhere in our environment. We may need to also take supplements that help to expel chemicals and heavy metals from our bodies. I suggest following the simple practice, outlined in this section, of selecting foods and modifying lifestyle habits to help expel heavy metals, as well as protect us from being overly exposed.

Plastics: After studies and news reports on the dangers of BPA, manufacturers began to produce BPA-free plastics, but new studies showed they still had a toxin called BPS which was just as harmful. It mimics estrogen just like BPA and interferes with the way cells respond to existing estrogen. It changes cell growth patterns even in tiny doses. Researchers found that 93 percent of the Americans they tested had BPS in the urine!

Chemicals: Another research study tested a group of families for man-made toxins and every single person in each family from the youngest to the oldest had toxins like PCBs, organochlorine pesticides (insecticides, solvents and fumigants are highly toxic and have negative effects on your central nervous system, CNS)[56], brominated flame retardants, and perfluorinated chemicals (used in carpet treatments to resist stains and water, however, has reproductive, developmental and systemic effects on humans and animals.)[57]. The U.S. Centres for Disease Control found 148 chemicals in the blood and urine samples of 2,400 Americans. More than a quarter of the samples contained beno(a)pryene, a toxin found in exhaust fumes.[58] I can go on and on with all the scientific research findings, but I think you understand the seriousness of what is going on with our exposure to chemicals.

MERCURY

Mercury is found in so many places that it is not hard to have exposure to it. It is found in such things as air conditioning filters, adhesives, cosmetics, fabric softener, laxatives, tattoos, seafood, vaccinations, and in the air as well. The mercury from coal-fired power plants is floating in the air. Silver dental amalgam fillings are a main source of contamination. They contain 50 percent mercury and can be poisonous to the body. Their particles and vapor are being continuously released as you chew, grind and brush your teeth. Therefore, it is important to get them removed. Unfortunately, mercury is also found in many of our fish. Swordfish and king mackerel have high levels of mercury, therefore should rarely be eaten. Tuna steaks and canned tuna also have mercury concentrations; however, the ones packed in water have less. Pregnant women and children should avoid seafood with high levels of mercury. Use omega-3 fish oil supplements without mercury, dioxins, and polychlorinated biphenyls also known as PCBs (an industrial compound used in electrical equipment, transformers and capacitors that when accumulated in animal tissue can become pathogenic.)[59]

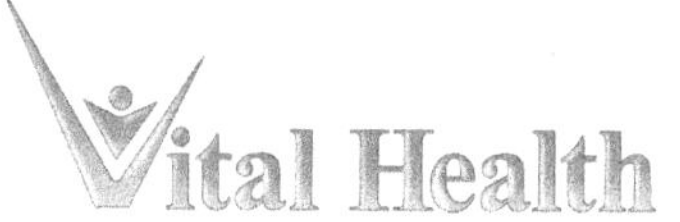

LEAD

Lead is poisonous even in tiny amounts. This heavy metal is stored in your kidneys, liver, brain, teeth and bones. It is unavoidable because it's in the soil and water supply. Children who absorb more lead than adults can experience behavioral challenges and reduction in IQ. Some of the ways to limit lead exposure are: don't use lead paint, take shoes off when entering your home so you don't track soil which has lead in it, get water filters for tap water. There are many good water filter systems out there. One that I have found easy to use is by BelKraft. They are portable and fasten to your tap kitchen faucets. A four-stage ceramic cartridge removes bacteria, heavy metals, chlorine and toxic chemicals from the tap water. The water becomes alkaline balanced, keeping the minerals that we need still in the water. You can go to Belkraft.com to check out the different type of filters they provide. They are also reasonably priced at around a few hundred dollars. You only have to replace the filters every 18 months or so. The number to call is 613-523-7800 or email ron@belkraft.com. In the meantime, if you don't have a filter, run your taps for a few minutes if they haven't been used for a few hours. In addition, use cold water for cooking and drinking because hot water leaches lead from the pipes.

ALUMINUM

This is another substance to avoid. Aluminum has been linked to Alzheimer's disease, memory problems, strokes and heart attacks. One of the main commercial products you want to avoid is antiperspirants which use Aluminum Zirconium which glue your sweat glands closed. This will prevent toxins from being removed and have been linked to a higher incidence of breast cancer.

WHAT TO DO?

Heavy metal cleanse products: Advanced Bionutritionals has an effective heavy-metal cleanse product called PectaSol made from citrus pectin, the inner peel of citrus fruits, and alginates made from seaweed. Both are made of soluble fibres that trap toxins in the stomach, circulate through the bloodstream and trap toxic metal ions like lead, mercury, cadmium and arsenic to eliminate them. Take as prescribed for the period of time instructed. Many companies offer all kinds of heavy metal cleanse products. It's best to try the products of one company first and see how you feel and how it works for you and then decide which ones are best for your body and needs. I suggest you start with this company because it was referred to me by an expert on top quality food-based supplements. Visit Advanced Bionutritionals at www.advancedbionutritionals.com. If you are ordering from Eastern part of Canada give at least 6 weeks or more for shipping.

Chelation therapy: This is the introduction of chelating agents that bind and remove heavy metals from the body. Your body does naturally chelate these heavy metals. However, with increasing pollution and toxicity levels, your body can't eliminate it all and it begins to accumulate. Fortunately, there are a few economical supplements like PectaSol, as mentioned earlier, that can help your body expel these unwanted toxins.

CILANTRO

Cilantro is also known as Chinese parsley or coriander. It is a natural herb and an effective natural chelator of toxic metal accumulated in the nervous system, bones and body tissues. Research shows cilantro can bind to heavy metals and flush them from the body. It has a wonderful taste and can be used fresh in many recipes such as soups and salads. You can take fresh cilantro, cilantro tincture or cilantro tea. The most economical and enjoyable way to use cilantro is to make a

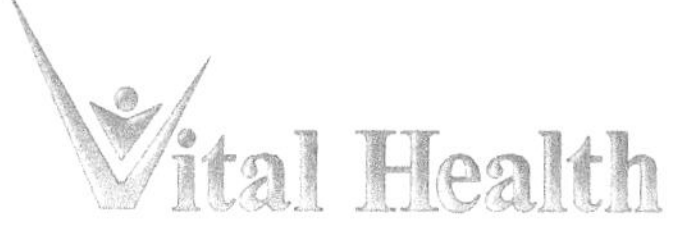

batch of fresh cilantro pesto and take 2 teaspoons a day for 3 weeks to flavor your food. Add it to pasta, vegetables, chicken, fish, beef dishes and even just bread. It's so versatile!

A simple recipe for Cilantro pesto:

Ingredients:

- 1 clove garlic
- ½ cup almonds, walnuts, pine nuts or other nuts
- 1 cup packed fresh cilantro leaves
- 2 tbsp lemon juice
- 6 tbsp olive oil

Add all ingredients into a food processor and blend. This recipe can be doubled and tripled and then refrigerated for a few days. You can even put it in the freezer in ice cube trays.

CHLORELLA

Chlorella is a type of algae that has numerous health benefits, including boosting the immune system and protecting the body from bacteria and viruses. It contains protein and antioxidants, and boosts energy levels by increasing the oxygen level in the blood. It is also very effective in cleansing the body of these burdensome heavy metals.

Chlorella works by binding to the heavy metals and other environmental toxins, acting as a sponge to remove them from the body. When taken in conjunction with cilantro, it works even better than when taken alone. It can be found in powder and tablet form. Generally, it's best to take chlorella 30 minutes after cilantro. This is because cilantro mobilizes the heavy metals, and then chlorella absorbs and eliminates them.

VITAMIN C

Vitamin C supports the body's detoxification process. It helps protect your immune system from the mobilized toxins as they leave your body. Take 1,000 mg of Vitamin C daily, after meals and separately from chlorella.

GARLIC

Garlic contains sulfur which is an excellent chelator of toxic metals such as mercury and lead. It oxidizes the heavy metals, making them water soluble and easy to excrete. You can add 2-3 fresh cloves a day to your food, otherwise look for reduced odor garlic tablets.[60]

Healthy Meal Plans

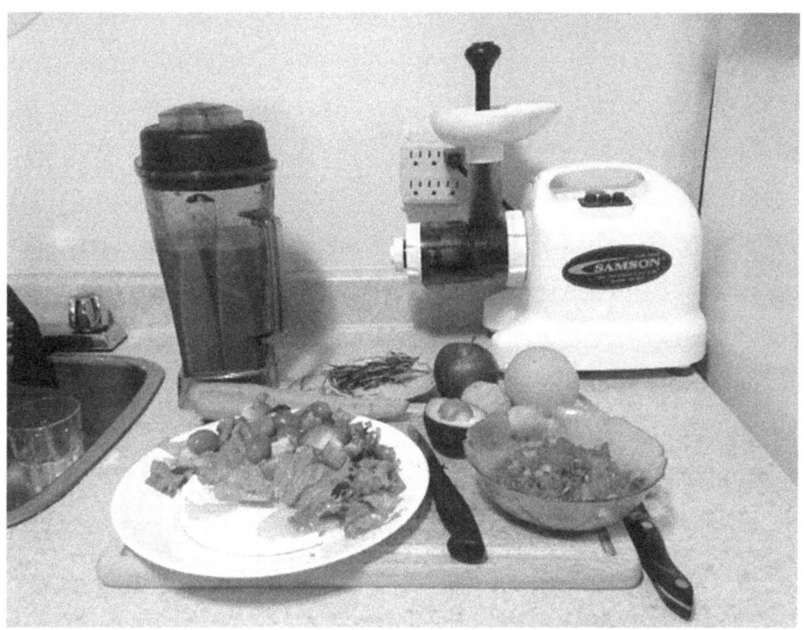

FOODS THAT KEEP THE HORMONES BALANCED

When you eliminate processed foods from your diet, it increases your body's frequencies. This makes you feel good because you will have greater mental clarity to think and carry out your daily tasks. We are basically made out of atoms which translate to energy. Furthermore, when you take the time to make a healthy meal for yourself and your family, it causes you to live in the moment and allows you to be focused, in a state of meditation, where you are just working with the organic foods and creating a meal. It really helps you to de-stress from the day's demands.

Try as much as possible to buy organic produce and fruits that are otherwise high on the chemical spray list when not organic. Here is a list of the produce and fruits that are highly sprayed:

Apples (worst)
Celery (worst)
Strawberries (worst)
Peaches
Spinach
Nectarines
Grapes
Sweet bell peppers
Potatoes
Blueberries
Lettuce
Kale/ Collards

If you cannot always get organic, then use a wash mixture that will remove some of the chemicals off vegetables like carrots, tomatoes and apples. You can make your own homemade solution of 1 tbsp lemon, 2 tbsp white vinegar and 1 cup of filtered water. Put this in a spray bottle and spray produce and hard fruits, rub for 30 seconds and rinse with purified water.[61]

- Frozen vegetables and fruits are better than fresh non-organic if they are on the high spray list.
- Try to buy organic, free-range meat, poultry, wild fish and dairy products from organically fed cows, goats and chickens. Stay away from non-organic chicken, turkey, pork or beef as much as possible. These tend to have high amounts of hormones and toxins, especially if they are coming from huge grocery chains in the United States. Avoid all deli-processed meats. Limit consumption of large fish such as swordfish, tuna, and sole due to high levels of mercury. Also, entirely avoid farmed salmon because of the high toxins. Keep your intake of high saturated fat, meats, and full-fat dairy products and safflower and sunflower oils to less than 50 percent of your weekly intake of meats, dairy and oils.
- Use cold-pressed olive oil and sesame oil which is very high in zinc. Zinc promotes collagen production for bone and healthy skin. It is also high in magnesium which has been shown to lower blood pressure in diabetics.[62]
- Consume 10 - 20 almonds, walnuts or pecans per day, (unless nut allergies are present).

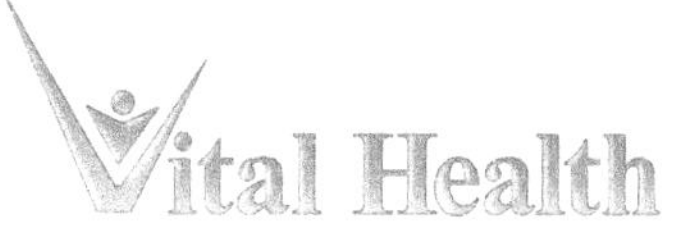

- Have a serving of beans every couple of days and take one to two scoops of non-flavoured whey isolate in a shake with some fruit every day.
- Have a minimum of 2 servings or more of fruit, like berries, pineapple, apples, pears, or other fruits. Always include one organic apple in the mix because of its high anti-oxidant value.
- Don't worry about the calories as much as the quality of the food you are eating and pay attention to how you are combining your foods. Eat a portion size that is about the size of your fist. Try not to overeat at any given meal because it will increase stress in the body. Eat every 3 - 4 hours, this way your sugar levels are steady. If you are hungry at night before bed, stick to light fruit and a handful of nuts or a protein shake. If you are really hungry, then salad with chicken or tuna is a good choice. Also make sure you eat within an hour after a workout with higher amounts of carbohydrates than usual as you've used up quite a bit of sugars from the workout. Always eat before working out with weights, or you will fade fast.
- Stay away from foods that your body has allergic reactions to. Excess mucus after eating is usually a sign that your body is having a hard time dealing with that particular food. If you are not sure what you are allergic to, you can try eliminating all the foods that you think may be potential allergic foods for about 14 days. Then re-introduce each one back into your diet, one at a time, see how you feel and look for any visible symptoms and changes in how your body works.
- Entirely stay away from all foods sweetened with fructose, containing corn syrup, and artificial sweeteners since it elevates your appetite. Eighty percent of the time, stay away from raisins and dates because they are very high in sugar. However, you can minimize the sugar released by eating them with a protein shake or with nuts.

Stay away from non-organic coffee 80 percent of the time. If you really need it, have one organic coffee before your workout or before your lunch time so it doesn't interfere with your sleep. Also, if you use decaf, choose organic and Swiss water decaffeinated.[63]

These meal plans are all designed with foods that keep your body hormonally balanced and are non-inflammatory. Each snack and meal will be explained in the following pages and the meal plan for each type of need is seen in the daily meal plan sheets given. You can refer back and forth from the explanation sections to the actual meal sheets.

FOOD COMBINING

This is a topic worth mentioning because it will help a lot of you who have digestive issues, especially those of you who are struggling with acid reflux, bloating, gas and constipation. When you eat a protein such as meat, fish or chicken you should try as much as possible to eat it with some raw vegetables like a salad, steamed non-starchy vegetables or even a raw vegetable juice done in a juicer. The reason for this is because these vegetables are non-starchy, the body will not secrete the digestive enzymes for starchy foods at the same time it releases protein enzymes to breakdown the protein. Hence your digestion will take a lot less work on the digestive system and organs and the digestion of the food will only take about 3-4 hours. However, when we break this rule and eat meat with bread, pasta, rice or potatoes, the body releases both enzymes where they neutralize each other's effectiveness in breaking down the proteins and starchy food. Therefore, it takes about 12 hours to digest the meal and you may also feel more sluggish, experience acid indigestion, bloating, gas and constipation.

In a lot of cases the foods people consume in the western world are dry, dense with low water content. Foods like sandwiches, burgers and fries are typical examples of these kinds of foods. It would be better for you to wait about three hours after you consume a protein with a salad meal and have a separate carbohydrate meal of a potato with some salsa sauce on it. You will notice a significant difference in your digestion and energy level, because you are spending less energy digesting the food in your system and both digestive enzymes are not being released.

When it comes to fruits, they should be eaten alone because they only take about 20-30 minutes to digest. Then you can eat your main course of starchy food meal like whole wheat pasta, brown rice or potato or meat with steamed vegetables and salad. However, if you eat the fruit right after you eat the main course meal, you will possibly experience bloating, gas and some acid indigestion. This is because the fruit is digested quickly but because your stomach and small intestine is digesting the protein or starch for the three to four hours, the fruit starts to ferment and create a high acidic environment in your gut. Therefore, it's best to always eat your fruits about 30 minutes before the main course. You will notice a considerable difference in your digestion.

It's quite difficult to follow this food combining rule all the time, especially when you are traveling. I try to follow it about 50 percent of the time. One of the things that I do to help my system digest the food easier is I consume a glass of raw vegetable juice using such ingredients as carrots, kale, celery, beets and ginger. It really has a lot of raw enzymes that will make a difference in digesting the meal that you have not combined well. Also, I take extra probiotic before the meal which also makes a difference. Furthermore, drink plenty of water after the meal as well which also helps digestion. Another practice I do when I have ignored this rule is I drink another raw vegetable juice done fresh in a juicer about an hour or two after the meal with a few glasses of water. You may find that you will have a bowel movement after this and your stomach and system will feel much better, no more bloating or feeling of being backed up or constipated. For those of you suffering from chronic digestive issues like constipation, bloating and acid indigestion I suggest you follow the food combining rule over 80 percent with your meals. It will ease your digestive issues significantly. Also, taking a glass of raw vegetable juice once to twice a day with some probiotic will also make a difference. Please refer to the appendix chart at the back of the book on food combining.

HYDRATION

The first component of a healthy balanced meal plan starts with proper hydration. You should be taking in about three to six eight-ounce glasses of filtered water in the first hour and half of waking up in the morning. Since you have been sleeping for about eight hours and your system is dehydrated, you need to re-hydrate to get things moving and activate your digestive system.[64] This will help your body in its elimination cycle that lasts from 4 am to 12 pm. When you have eaten foods the night before that are low in water content, such as breads, pastas, meat and grains, you need more water to help digest these foods. So you may need to drink more than three glasses of water the next morning. In many cases, I find I need to drink about six to eight glasses of water in the morning. This activates a bowel movement to evacuate.[65]

Our bodies are about 70 percent water and our brain is about 80 percent water. We lose about 12 cups of water per day through sweat, urine and breathing. It is ESSENTIAL for us to replenish our body with water every day![66]

IMPORTANCE OF FRUITS

Fruits are a gentle simple sugar that produces less insulin response compared to complex carbohydrates like bread, potatoes, rice and pasta.[67] Full of enzymes, with a high water content and high in fibre, fruits are a great source of energy, especially when you are at a low point during the day.[68] This is due to the fact that fruits get digested very quickly in the stomach; usually about 30 minutes. Melons and kiwi take about 15-20 minutes. Their nutrients are released in the intestine more quickly than other fruits like apples, oranges, pears, etc. which take about 30 minutes to digest. Therefore, it's good to eat fruits in the morning on an empty stomach because fruits are digested completely in the stomach before moving on into the intestine. Watch your consumption of high fructose products like dried raisins, dates, honey, raw sugar, agave, molasses, maple syrup, and sucanat. High fructose food consumption increases uric acid which leads to inflammation that can lead to inflamed blood vessels causing heart attacks and strokes. Also, the high uric acid levels in the body causes nitric oxide to decrease, raising angiotensin causing the smooth muscle cells to contract, raising blood pressure and eventually damaging kidneys. I would keep it to a teaspoon every few days. [69]

The water soluble vitamins like Vitamin C, most of the B vitamins, the minerals and the fat soluble vitamins of the fruit will be readily absorbed when the leftover fruit fibre goes into the small intestine. This is why it is crucial to wait 30 minutes before eating breakfast so that the digestion of the fruit is not hindered.[70]If you eat fruit after consuming cooked protein or carbohydrates or both, the fruit will digest much sooner than both of these foods[71]. As other foods are digested, the fruit will begin to ferment, along with any carbohydrates and proteins. It takes about three hours for starchy vegetables to digest; meats take about four hours;

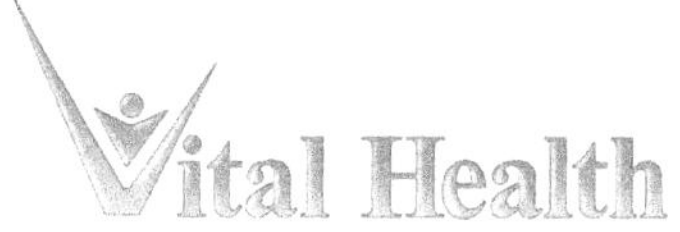

fish and chicken about three hours. The end result is the stomach becomes acidic, leading to chronic acid indigestion problems and use of antacids.[72]

Eating starchy carbohydrates, like potatoes, rice and pasta, with protein will also affect digestion. The enzymes that digest carbohydrates and proteins and the acids that digest the protein neutralize one another. A meal of protein and starchy carbohydrates will take about 12 hours to digest, instead of three hours.[73]

BREAKFAST TIME

Breakfast A, which focuses on whole grain cereals like quinoa, millet, oatmeal or a seed cereal, is for those who don't need a heavy, large breakfast. The first three cereals are basically carbohydrates that contain some protein.

Quinoa, which actually comes from the fruit family, is low in gluten and high in protein and has all the essential amino acids. Quinoa is an excellent source of phosphorus, Vitamin E, and many B vitamins. It is the least mucus forming and is high in calcium. A cup of quinoa is equal to a quart of milk in calcium.

Millet is another ancient low-gluten grain, high in vitamins, minerals, rich in phosphorus, calcium, iron, niacin and riboflavin. Also it's low in calories; one cup is only 90 calories.

Oats have soluble fibre that can help lower cholesterol levels and work at keeping the colon healthy. Whole oats may take longer to cook, but are high in nutrients with seven B vitamins, Vitamin E, nine minerals, calcium and iron.

The **seed cereal** is basically a raw protein cereal with omega oils which makes it a very high nutrient food. It is also a non-inflammatory food. Because it is not cooked, the nutrients in the seeds are not destroyed. This is the same seed cereal recipe given in the previous cleanse recipe sheet for juicing and protein shakes. This seed cereal recipe was developed by my mentor in health, Julian Beecroft, who was my father figure and worked until he was nearly 97 and lived till nearly 100.

SEED CEREAL NUTRIENT SUMMARY:

Flax Seeds: high in oil which is high in EFAs, fibre, protein and mucilage which absorbs toxins and lubricates;

Sunflower Seeds: 22% protein, contain 50% oil, high in iron and 7 mgs per 100 milligrams of seeds; high in Potassium which helps reduce sodium in the body; contains linoleic acid which reduces cholesterol deposits in the arteries and veins; High in magnesium and phosphorus;

Pumpkin Seeds: high source of Vitamin A, iron, Vitamin B1, B2 and B3;

Sesame Seeds: 19% protein, high source of B vitamins, calcium and minerals; best to eat the ones with the husk on them because of the higher calcium content.[74]

FRESH JUICES

Freshly juiced vegetables and fruits have the enzymes, minerals and fine fibre equal to eating a bowl of salad, but is digested and absorbed more readily into the body. Fresh juices carry hundreds of micronutrients into the cells of the body to repair, heal and build. I suggest you have a tall 12-oz glass of a fresh, life-giving drink, full of micronutrients, every morning. The following lists the required portions of each ingredient and its nutritional makeup. The combination will make about four cups. If this is your first time juicing, try to keep to the required recipe quantity of each vegetable and fruit or you may end up with a strong flavour of one ingredient over the other. For example, if you put in a three-inch chunk of ginger root instead of just a one- or two-inch chunk, the juice mixture will have a dominant ginger flavour. It does not take much ginger to make the juice taste like ginger.

JUICE RECIPE VEGETABLES NUTRIENT SUMMARY:

8 to 12 carrots, depending on size, are high in calcium, Vitamin A, C, B complex, iron, potassium, phosphorus and sodium;

2 to 3 celery stalks are high in magnesium and iron, high in chlorophyll which is an excellent blood builder and rich in sodium which maintains body fluid and electrolytes when training;

1 small beet, or ¼ of a large one, contains calcium, sulfur, iron, potassium, choline, beta-carotene and Vitamin C which strengthen the liver, gall bladder and are building blocks for blood corpuscles and cells; and manganese which is important for brain function;

1 to 2 apples, based on size, have pectin that turns to gel in the intestine which helps to remove toxins in the bowels; apples also contain phosphorus and potassium which help flush the kidneys and calm the stomach; natural sugar develops acids which encourage saliva flow and digestion;

1 to 2-inch chunk of fresh ginger root is anti-bacterial, anti-viral and a digestive aid;

BREAKFAST A

- 1 tbsp omega-3 Oil or 3 gelatin capsules of Wild Salmon Oil
- One 50 mg Vitamin B complex capsule and 1 tsp of powdered Vitamin C
- 4 - 6 oz. protein seed cereal, organic oatmeal or millet cereal (Refer to seed cereal recipe p. 75)
- 6 - 8 oz of unsweetened almond milk, goat's milk or rice milk

- ½ tsp unpasteurized honey, sucanat (organic raw sugar) or maple syrup
- 8 - 12 oz. vegetable and fruit juice from juicer or green smoothie (Refer to Juice Recipe p. 77 or Smoothie Recipe p. 229)

Adding more protein: For people who need more calories and protein because their training is at a higher level of intensity and energy output, they can have Breakfast Sample A with Breakfast Sample B. Especially if you are trying to increase muscle size, strength and power as in serious bodybuilding, power lifting, shot-putting etc.

As long as there are no allergic reactions, eggs are one of the best sources of protein. They have one of the highest absorption rates compared to other protein foods, whereas other proteins like meats are actually less. Much of the fear surrounding eggs and cholesterol has been nullified by recent findings. In North America, many of the high cholesterol cases could be traced to people eating high saturated fatty foods like bacon, sausages and buttered toast with their eggs. While eggs may be high in cholesterol (186 milligrams, 184 of them in the yolk), they're relatively low in saturated fat (1.6 grams in the yolk)."[75] "The major determinant of plasma low-density lipoprotein (LDL, also known as the "bad fat") level is saturated fat," according to Alice Lichtenstein, professor of nutrition science and policy at the Friedman School of Nutrition Science and Policy at Tufts University. The lecithin in the egg yolk actually emulsifies the fat in the yolk so that it is broken down to smaller particles and more easily eliminated from the body.[76]

Also to really increase calories and muscle gain, I suggest having additional protein with your eggs, like an extra 4 oz. of canned tuna, salmon, sardines or leftover chicken and beef. Higher amounts of protein consumed per meal with adequate recovery time will increase your strength in the gym. Also when you take in enough quality carbohydrates with the protein, you will experience greater muscular endurance. Your muscles will feel tighter, fuller and your vascularity will be more noticeable. Hence, when you do a resistance exercise with a bar or dumbbell, the hypertrophy will be enhanced. This is that "pumped up feeling" that bodybuilders talk about.[77]

Tips on Training: Do not train on an empty stomach; you will need the energy to perform the exercises optimally. Always take in a protein or a carbohydrate meal within 45 minutes of your workout. This is important because of the quick breakdown of muscle tissue after a workout. I suggest a protein shake right after the workout to replenish, and then have a meal. For those who are doing lighter exercise programs, such as aerobic classes or floor work, I suggest you still take in a protein or vegetable-based protein shake right after the exercise session.

If you do not do heavy, intense training or exercise in a gym then having a boiled, poached egg or two should be enough for you at breakfast, along with the seed cereal. If you like oatmeal or other carbohydrate whole grain cereals, then have the eggs with some raw vegetables first for breakfast and then have the cereal about two hours or more later as a separate small meal or vice versa. This way you follow the food combining rule. Add almond milk, goat's milk or rice milk to your cereal with a teaspoon of honey, a few drops of liquid stevia or maple syrup and it should be a satisfying small midmorning snack or meal. It will take some time to get used to this way of eating your meals, but you will find that your digestion will be 100% better, unhindered hormones, and a body free of inflammation.

NUTRITIOUS COMPONENTS OF A MEAL

Watch how you combine: It's important, as much as possible, to eat a raw vegetable salad or lightly steamed vegetables with your meat, chicken or fish protein. Non-starchy vegetables have a high-water content and can be digested in any type of digestive juices. They combine well with protein and will help digest protein in about three to four hours instead of the 12 hours or more when protein is combined with starchy carbohydrates.[78]

Mixing your salad: On your salads, use first cold-pressed oils like olive oil, avocado oil, hemp oil or organic sesame oil. Unfortunately, oils commonly used in restaurants or in store-bought salad dressings usually have been heated at higher temperatures and processed multiple times, thereby decreasing the nutrient value of the oil. “First cold-pressed” isn’t an official designation for olive oil. It basically means the fruit of the olive was crushed exactly one time, i.e., the “first press.” The “cold” refers to the temperature range of the fruit at the time it’s crushed. The temperature during this process is kept around 86 degrees Fahrenheit.[79]

Lemon is a healthy choice because it becomes alkaline after digestion in the body helping the body stay in a more alkaline state. It’s first acidic in your mouth as you are chewing, but becomes alkaline after digestion.[80] Balsamic vinegar has properties which combat heart disease and the polyphenols help in absorption of amino acids for building and repairing cells.[81]

Parsley is another great addition to meals which is high in anti-oxidants, vitamins, minerals, and fibre. It is both a food and a medicinal herb. It helps control blood-cholesterol, prevents constipation and protects the body from free radicals. It also contains oil called Eugonal used by dentists as a local anesthetic and antiseptic for tooth and gum disease. It’s used in many Mediterranean dishes and can be added in salads as a fresh spice. You can use Italian or flat leaf parsley.[82] It’s also best to choose organic since regular grocery store parsley can be highly sprayed. A similar plant that I enjoy is cilantro which looks like parsley, but has differently shaped leaves. They both belong to the plant family of Umbelliferae. Cilantro is also known as a Chinese parsley and is considered both a herb and a spice. It is full of phytonutrients and anti-oxidants. Its leaves and seeds contain essential oils. It also can be used as a natural anti-septic, analgesic, aphrodisiac, digestive aid and fungicide. A good source of vitamins A, C, and K, cilantro carries a high amount of calcium, potassium, iron, manganese and sodium. There is an antibiotic compound called Dodecenal isolated from cilantro which is just as effective as Gentamicin which kills food-borne bacteria salmonella.[83] Also the high amount of anti-oxidants in cilantro such as beta carotene, Vitamin C, E, kaempferol and quercetin have been linked to helping lower the risk of cancer causing cells in the body.[84]

Hummus is a Middle Eastern dip made from chick peas, olive oil, garlic, lemon juice and tahini (a sesame seed paste). It is a good source of non-meat protein with vitamins, minerals and high unsaturated fat. You can add it to salads because it helps make the salad more filling.[85]

BREAKFAST B

This breakfast consists of two boiled or poached eggs or two to three scrambled eggs or an omelette made in a non-stick, non-Teflon coated pan with a tablespoon of olive oil.

(Note: For athletes who need more calories and are trying to gain more muscle size, add 4 oz. tuna, salmon, beef, or chicken with the eggs, and an 8 to 12 oz. protein shake.)

With the eggs, have a bowl of salad with a tablespoon of olive oil, lemon juice or balsamic vinegar, sea salt, black pepper, parsley or cilantro and 1 to 2 oz. of hummus.

Vitamin B complex supplement: A Vitamin B complex needs to be taken regularly; every day or every other day. One of the main reason you take extra supplements of Vitamin B is they are water soluble and the body uses them up quickly and does not store it. Your body can only store a certain amount of the B vitamins so it needs to be replenished regularly. Water soluble vitamins like B and C are absorbed in the digestive tract into the blood stream and metabolized. Then it is excreted by the kidneys in the urine.[86] Thiamine, B1 in food is not that stable and can be destroyed by cooking and processing of any kind. Therefore it's essential to take a Vitamin B complex in the diet. Powder form is the best because it has about a 25 percent absorption rate whereas tablets are usually only five to 10 percent. [87] You need to take 50 mg to 100 mg capsules of Vitamin B complex. Some of the brands I use are Natural Factors and Sisu. You can usually get it in powder form in these brands. Take one powdered capsule a day with or after breakfast. If you are losing a lot of body water from long distance running, intense sport or competing in bodybuilding or fitness physique shows then take two capsules per day, one in the morning and evening during the high training periods. A more detailed breakdown of each of the B vitamins and what each one does in the body is given in the Supplements section near the end of the book.[88]

Vitamin C supplement: Vitamin C is another water soluble vitamin and is one of the most important vitamins for the body's immune system. Again, powdered form is better because it's about 25 percent absorption, whereas tablet form is around five to 10 percent absorption.[89] Take a level teaspoon of this with breakfast.

- 1 - 2 tsp per day (approx. 1500 to 3000 mg)
- Take ½ to 1 tsp with 2 oz. juice or water with or after breakfast.
- Take a second ½ - 1 tsp with 2 oz. water or juice with or after supper.

Vitamin C combined with Lysine helps make collagen stronger which can help prevent coronary attacks. This is a water-soluble vitamin, one of the most important for the immune system. It's necessary for absorption of iron, production of stress hormones and helps wounds to heal. It is also involved with growth and repair of blood vessels, cells, gums, bones and teeth.[90]

There are two products I personally use that I have found to aid in digestion, cleansing and keeps my immune system high, the first is a liquid vitamin called Daily Complete that I recommend which has 194 organic ingredients, with minerals, vitamins, herbs, phytoplankton, organic vegetables, fruits, enzymes and seeds. It is gluten free with a 60 percent absorption rate. It is also listed in the 2011 Compendium of Pharmaceuticals & Specialties that doctors and pharmacists refer to. Take two level tablespoons straight up or mix with water. It has a nice fruity taste. The second product is a naturally formulated Mediterranean cleansing product called Experience which helps promote regularity, digestion, breaks down gall and kidney stones, cleanses your digestive system and eventually the other systems of the body. It is made from ingredients like psyllium seed husk, senna leaf, fennel, kelp and rhubarb root. Both of these products are made by a company called Pure Trim. If you want to try this product, see the instruction sheet that was provided in the previous juice cleanse section. The founder of the company is Marc Tahiliani, N.D. You can learn more about these products at vitalcleanse.puretrim.com.

Experience can be taken in the evening or before bed as one capsule with a glass of water or you can also open up the capsule and pour the herbal powder into about five ounces of warm water and take as a tea. Add a half teaspoon of organic molasses which makes it alkaline and gives it a nice taste. You should notice some cleansing reactions by the body the next morning, such as more frequent bowel movements, some watery stool, diarrhea, gas, etc. If you don't notice

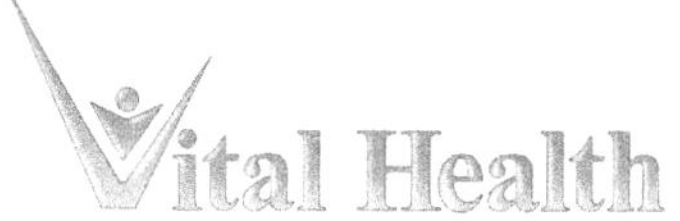

anything, then increase to two capsules the next evening. That should be enough to work. If there is still no cleansing reactions after two capsules, then increase to three, and if necessary, to four. I have encountered some people with highly toxic systems who needed to activate the cleansing action of the herbs by taking up to four to five capsules at the beginning. However, most only need up to two capsules.

MID-MORNING SNACK

I recommend a protein shake for a snack. You can use a non-flavoured whey isolate protein with some fruit if you like. However, if you want top quality, I suggest a vegetarian shake called Pure Trim made from about 70 live food sources including fermented vegetables. For those of you who are training with weights and are looking for additional protein, I recommend adding an extra scoop or two of non-flavoured whey isolate with half a pack of Pure Trim. If you are leaning down on a weight loss program, just the Pure Trim shake works well and has over 20 g of protein which is enough. The recipe on how to make a shake is on the products instruction sheet in the previous cleansing section under Pure Trim Products Instructions.

LUNCH

- Drink 1 to 2 cups of filtered water before the meal
- Choose either 4 - 6 oz of chicken, seafood, turkey, beef, or lean lamb (you can marinate for 15 minutes or longer with thyme, black pepper, sea salt, garlic, chopped onion, ½ oz of rice vinegar, ½ oz of sherry and 2 tbsp of organic barbeque sauce)
- Add either 8 - 12 oz of broccoli, Brussell sprouts, green beans, kale, cauliflower, etc., with a ¼ tsp of sea salt, ground pepper, ½ tsp of butter and sprinkle some roasted sesame seeds on it.
- Make sure you also have 12 oz or more of garden salad made of romaine lettuce, cucumbers, celery, green or bell pepper, tomatoes, fresh cilantro or parsley,

shredded carrots and 1 tbsp olive oil & balsamic or lemon juice. You also want to drink at least 1 - 2 cups of filtered water with the meal to hydrate.

You can marinate proteins such as chicken, turkey, fish, lean beef or lamb in some spices, fresh garlic, wine, a tablespoon of organic barbeque sauce and rice vinegar. Of course it's best to bake, barbeque, broil or steam your meats to minimize the fat content. Another condiment that can be used on meat is tomato chutney or hamburger relish. Look for home-made relish at local butchers or specialty deli shops. Again the selection of vegetables to have with the meat can be any two of these vegetables: steamed broccoli; green beans; cauliflower; collards; swiss chard; spinach or cabbage. The vegetables can be seasoned with a tablespoon of olive oil, a teaspoon of low sodium tamari sauce, 1/4 teaspoon of ground black pepper, sea salt and a teaspoon of roasted sesame seeds on top.

Sea salt is a better choice than table salt because there is less processing involved and contains potassium, magnesium and calcium. It is basically made from evaporated sea-water. However, you still need to be aware of how much you are consuming because the sodium content is the same as table salt at 40 percent.[91]

With the protein and steamed vegetables, you should have a serving of raw salad of your choice with fresh lemon juice squeezed or balsamic vinegar, sprinkled with sea salt and pepper or whatever spices you'd like to put on the salad. If you have high blood pressure, keep your daily sodium intake to around 1500 mg

Table 1: Recommended intake for sodium

HEALTHY...	SHOULD AIM FOR THE ADEQUATE INTAKE (AI) OF	WITHOUT GOING OVER THE UPPER LIMIT (UL) OF
Infants 0-6 months	120 mg/day	No data
Infants 7-12 months	370 mg/day	No data
Children 1-3 years	1000 mg/day	1500 mg/day
Children 4-8 years	1200 mg/day	1900 mg/day
Teens 9-13 years	1500 mg/day	2200 mg/day
Adults 14-50 years	1500 mg/day	2300 mg/day
Older adults 51-70 years	1300 mg/day	
Older adults over 70 years	1200 mg/day	
Pregnancy	1500 mg/day	

(http://www.hc-sc.gc.ca/fn-an/nutrition/sodium/index-eng.php#a2, Health Canada)

MID-NOON SNACKS OR MEAL

Drink one to two cups of water before or during a small meal or snack

(Note: You can have one, two or three of these suggestions as a snack or as a mid-noon meal based on your activity level and hunger.)

- 4 - 8 oz plain organic yogurt with 1 oz of raw or unsalted roasted nuts
- 4 - 8 oz. pineapple or other fruits with ¼ tsp of cinnamon and unsweetened almond milk
- 4 - 12 oz or more of potato/yam, squash, brown rice, whole wheat pasta, vermicelli noodles or soba buckwheat noodles
- 8 - 14 oz protein shake

For a snack at mid-noon, if you are not too hungry, about 4 - 8 oz. fresh fruit will be sufficient. You can mix some apples or berries with banana. Sprinkle it with cinnamon and pour on some almond milk. Almond milk is a good alternative to milk; a cup of almond milk has one gram of fibre and protein and is about 30 to 40 calories. It has about two to three grams of unsaturated fat. It is a safe drink for people with heart disease. It contains omega-3 fatty acids which can lower bad cholesterol. This healthy drink also contains significant amounts of magnesium, selenium, manganese and Vitamin E. Magnesium is involved in converting food to energy, aids the parathyroid glands that produce hormones that promote good bone health. Manganese is a mineral that activates enzymes that help digestion and also helps keep teeth and bones strong. Selenium supports the immune system as well.

If you need to have more food, a complex carbohydrate meal at mid-noon is a good habit to stick to. If you are planning to train after work or in the early evening this will get your glycogen levels up in your muscles. Therefore, this allows the muscles to work during your anaerobic activity. A quick complex carbohydrate recipe I consume regularly is 8 - 12 oz. of brown rice. I add a tablespoon of sesame oil, ½ tsp of tamari sauce, roasted sesame seeds with 2 - 4 oz of kimchi or sauerkraut. Brown rice is one of those carbohydrates that contain a starch called amylose which slows down the digestive process of the rice which allows for blood sugar levels to be more stable. Rice is one of the most nutritious grains. A pound of rice delivers four times the food energy than the same serving of potatoes or pasta. It is 80 percent starch and is a good source of protein, thiamin, phosphorus and carbohydrate. One cup of uncooked rice has 700 calories. About 8 oz of steamed rice has about 50 g of carbohydrate.

A good topping for any whole grain pasta dish can include some tomato sauce made from the following ingredients: a few garlic cloves minced, ½ ounce of fresh parsley and cilantro chopped, one chopped celery stalk, one slice sweet Spanish onion cooked in a tablespoon of olive oil and red wine. Pour this sauce on top of the pasta with some grated mozzarella cheese and you have a fine carb meal.

Whole wheat pasta has more health benefits. It is higher in fibre, natural bran, germ, vitamins and minerals. Normal white pasta does not have these traits because it's been processed. Because of the higher fibre, whole wheat pasta makes you feel full faster and it promotes better bowel movements. Whole wheat pasta also contains iron, B vitamins, selenium, magnesium and folic acid. If there is gluten intolerance and allergy to wheat, try buckwheat which is low in gluten or vermicelli noodles which is rice based. You can buy these in Asian food stores. They are lighter and easier to digest and a good choice if you don't want too much starch in your meals. I personally consume mostly buckwheat, whole wheat soba and rice noodles. You can also buy organic whole grain pasta at the health food stores.

A sweet potato or normal white potato is a good choice as a complex carbohydrate meal. You can put an ounce of salsa or tsaziki on it for flavor or both as a topping. If you need something fast and easily digestible then a protein shake is also an option. The normal potatoes like Yukon Gold are a good source of Vitamin C, potassium, calcium and iron. The most nutritious part is the skin. They also are high in starch. Red potatoes are less starchy and lower in calories. The best kind of potato is the ones with eyes, meaning they are ready to sprout. This also means they are high in enzymes. Sweet potatoes, on the other hand, have a high amount of beta carotene. They are also high in Vitamin C, potassium, calcium and fibre. The potato family are all complex carbohydrates, meaning they are made of long complex chains of simple sugars and are slower to digest, converting into sugars and raising blood sugar levels. However, starches that have been processed, turn into sugar very rapidly in the body and have a higher glycemic index.

PROTEIN SUPPLEMENTS

Vital Health Protein Shake Recipes:

- 2 scoops of unflavored whey isolate or whey concentrate powder
- ½ pack of Pure Trim shake (Mediterranean meal replacement)
- 2 ½ cups of filtered water
- 1 banana
- 4-6 oz. frozen strawberries or other kinds of fruits
- 1-2 oz. unsweetened almond or goat's milk (optional for a more creamy texture)

Whey Protein

The main reasons whey protein is used:

- Convenient because you can prepare it quicker than foods like meats, fish, dairy, and eggs
- Contain a lot less fat and cholesterol found in high protein foods
- Cheaper than most protein foods like beef and fish
- Supplies more protein
- Great tasting and can be used by the whole family

There are two kinds of protein powders: animal source and vegetable source. Animal source is made from whey, casein, goat's milk and egg white protein. Vegetable source come from soy, rice, pea and hemp proteins. Whey protein is the most commonly used, but soy protein from the vegetable source is also used. The protein portion of whole milk is 20 percent whey protein and 80 percent casein protein. There are two types of whey:

Whey concentrate and whey isolate. Whey concentrate has low lactose levels and some fat and carbs. Whey isolate is virtually fat free, lactose free and has a thinner consistency.

Casein Protein

Casein is another milk protein used, but releases slower in the digestive system compared to whey protein. It's labeled usually as calcium caseinate.

Egg White Protein

Egg white protein is a popular protein type. It tastes good. It's also low in fat, carbs and cholesterol free. It's a good alternative for those wanting non-dairy protein. Fitness Labs sells a brand called Egg Fit Protein.

Vegetable Proteins

Soy and hemp protein is popular. They both supply all eight essential amino acids, most vegetable proteins lack one or more. Unfortunately, there are some studies showing negative effects of the isoflavone in soya, where estrogen-dependent tumor growth increased as the soy diet increased. Hemp is a safer choice.

However, a clean vegetable protein that has the least amount of issues is organic pea and brown rice protein. Brown rice protein has all of the nine essential amino acids and is considered a complete protein. It is low in heavy metals and they have been able to separate it from the grain and starch component of the rice. Therefore, it is gluten free. Studies have shown it to aid in muscle recovery, gains in muscle, and increase in strength. It has minimal allergic effects compared to milk proteins. In addition, pea protein combined with rice protein is very effective because rice protein is high in the amino acids methionine and cysteine, but low in lysine. However, pea protein is high in lysine so when combined, these two proteins are really good alternatives to whey protein. Methionine helps to diminish muscle weakness. Cysteine promotes the burning of fat in the body and the building of muscle. Lysine works with the other amino acids to maintain growth, lean body mass and the body's store of nitrogen. A deficiency in this amino acid can result in fatigue, lack of concentration, irritability, bloodshot eyes, retarded growth, hair loss, anaemia and reproductive challenges.

Studies have shown we lose about .5 to 2 percent of muscle from the age of 45 on. The main reason is from not enough digested protein in the diet. This is why I am a huge promoter of having high amounts of protein in the diet for everyone.

I use an organic pea and brown rice protein called Pure Trim, found at vitalcleanse.puretrim.com. It can be used as a meal replacement or as a supplement between meals. It is based on the Mediterranean diet where they eat olive oil, unrefined grains, nuts, seeds, fish and vegetables. The shake powder itself is a combination of protein complex of non-GMO vegetable pea protein concentrate and brown rice protein.

PURE TRIM INGREDIENTS:

Mediterranean essential fatty acid blend of safflower oil, almond oil, flax seed, grape seed, olive and sesame oils; **Prebiotic and Enzyme blend** bromelain, acacia, inulin, lipase and protease; ionic plant trace mineral blend (ocean plant); **Anti stress and Energy blend** of green tea leaf extract, passion flower, cinnamon twig extract, galangal root extract, ginseng, peppermint, rhodiola root extract, mate leaf extract; **Mediterranean Skin & Digestive blend** of Olive leaf extract, artichoke leaf extract, grape leaf, pomegranate fruit extract. **Super Greens Blend**: alfalfa leaf, asparagus, spear extract, barley grass, bitter lemon fruit extract, broccoli floret, Brussels sprout leaf, cabbage leaf, cauliflower floret, chlorella, mustard seed, nettle leaf, spirulina, cocoa bean, sea salt, silica, acesulfame potassium, sucralose, stevia leaf extract.

Also the calcium from this shake is from plant sources instead of from calcium carbonate which is same as limestone used in cement.

GOAT'S MILK

Goat's milk is a very digestible dairy product because the molecular size is similar to composition of human mother's milk. Any species of mammal can be raised on goat's milk. It provides 13 percent more calcium, 25 percent more Vitamin B6, 47 percent more Vitamin A, 134 percent more potassium and 350 percent more niacin than cow's milk. Also goat's milk requires no homogenization because the fat droplets in goat's milk are about 20 percent the size of cow milk's fat droplets and they remain evenly dispersed in the liquid portion of the milk. Studies show the consumption of homogenized milk can lead to atherosclerosis.

You can absorb goat's milk in about 20 minutes, but it takes about two to three hours to digest cow's milk. Goat's milk also increases the PH level in the blood stream because it has a high amounts of the amino acid glutamine which is an alkalizing amino acid. It does not produce mucus or worsen allergic respiratory conditions such as asthma. Goat's milk has been known to have anti-inflammatory and prebiotic effects on the digestive system.

The August 2001 issue of the *Journal of Dairy Research* reports a study comparing cow and goat milk. It was found that compared with cow milk, goat milk reduced cholesterol levels. It was also found that goat milk fat was more easily absorbed in rats that had parts of their intestines removed, and therefore was more tolerated than cow's milk. The digestive utilization of goat milk was compared to that of olive oil. From these observations, the authors note that goat's milk can be useful in patients with certain intestinal problems, especially persons who have undergone intestinal surgery. Goat's milk contains twice the healthful medium-chain fatty acids, such as capric and caprylic acids, which are highly antimicrobial. Goat's milk has a higher concentration of medium chain fatty acids which play an important role in imparting unique health benefits. Medium chain fatty acids minimize cholesterol deposition in the arteries, aid in dissolving cholesterol and gallstones, and significantly contribute to normal growth of infants.

SUPPER

- Drink 1 to 2 cups of filtered water before the meal
- Have a bowl of organic vegetable soup, i.e. squash or roasted red pepper tomato soup. (note. store bought)
- Consume about 4 - 8 oz organic chicken, meat stew, beef, lamb, wild fresh fish or sea food. (note. stay away from large fish since they contain higher levels of heavy metals)
- Combine this with 16 - 20 oz of non-starchy vegetables like broccoli, spinach, carrots, kale, Swiss chard, turnip, asparagus, green beans etc.
- In addition have 12 - 14 oz garden salad with 1 tbsp olive oil and lemon juice or seaweed salad.

Vital Health System's Seaweed Salad Recipe

- Soak about 4 large handful of dried seaweed in a bowl of boiled water for about 15 minutes
- Strain well and put into a mixing bowl
- Add two to three green onions chopped
- 1 - 2 garlic clove minced
- 1 lemon squeezed
- 2 - 3 tables of tamari sauce (low sodium, non-GMO, wheat free soya sauce)
- 1 tsp of raw or roasted sesame seeds
- 2 tbsp of sesame oil
- 1 tsp of raw brown sugar (optional)
- Mix well and serve with some fish and steamed vegetables or with steamed brown rice and some pickled, fermented vegetables like Kimchi and Dai Kong (pickled Japanese radish)

Organic Chicken

Organic chicken minimizes the risk of exposure to antibiotics and pesticides in the feed. Also, there is less risk in harmful bacteria that are found in meat produced in confined animal feeding operations. Lean organic chicken is a low fat protein and a good source of selenium, zinc, niacin, vitamin E, beta-carotene, and vitamin B6 and B12. Meat from chicken allowed access to the outdoors has 21 percent less total fat, 30 percent less saturated fat, 28 percent less calories, 50 percent more vitamin A, and 100 percent more omega-3 fatty acid than chickens that are not allowed outdoors.

(USDA Sustainable Agriculture & Research Education Program)

Organic Beef

Organic grass-fed beef is what you want to consume. Here are some of the reasons.

Grass-fed beef only has 10 percent saturated fat verses non-grass-fed beef which is about 50 percent saturated fat. Also the omega-3 from the grass fed cows is two to four times higher and is very nutritious; higher in good unsaturated fats and lower in bad saturated fats. The meat is three to five times higher in conjugated linoleic acid (CLA). It has 400 percent more Vitamin A (as beta-carotene) and E.

There is no risk of Mad Cow Disease. Six ounces of this kind of beef also has 100 less calories than 6 oz of grain-fed beef.

Farmed vs. Wild Fish

As much as possible, consume wild fish. So much of the fish commercially available comes from fish farms. I think this article from oneresult.com will explain why you should buy only fresh or wild fish.

"Wild salmon are like the equivalent of local, grass fed beef from a small farm. Unfortunately only 10 - 20% of the US salmon supply comes from the wild. The other 80% is farmed. Fish farming, aka aquaculture, has been called the equivalent of a "floating pig farm". Sick. But there are several other reasons why fish farming is processed meat nasty, besides being mean to poor little Nemo.

My man Dr. Seuss once said "One fish, two fish, red fish, and blue fish". How about grey fish? Yes, I'm talking about that distinguishing bright "pink" salmon flesh. What if it was actually an ugly grey that was dyed pink with synthetic pigments? No joke. You can even select which tone you want on your very own Salmon Farm! I wouldn't mind my kitchen being a #20 and my future (hybrid) Range Rover being a #33 or #34, but really, choosing the pigment of fish?

Wild salmon is naturally bright pink because it eats little pink krill (like mini shrimp). Farmed fish, on the other hand, eat ground up fish meal and fish oil – essentially processed food. Let's not even get into the use of genetically modified soy, vegetable protein, or chicken feathers and slaughter waste for food. Besides being unnatural, unsustainable, and polluting the environment, fish meal doesn't give those fishies the pretty pink color we're used to seeing. Enter the Salmon Farm. As if this wasn't already ridiculous enough, canthaxanthin, one of the most commonly used dyes, hasn't been proven safe and has been linked to vision damage. And that's just the beginning."[cxii]

Elk Meat

Elk is a healthier red meat choice to consume because of its leanness. It is about 3.3 percent fat per 25 g of a loin cut verses 9.7 g of fat for 31 g of round lean beef cut. Farmed elk is low in cholesterol and the ratio of polyunsaturated and monounsaturated fatty acids are higher than in our common red meat selections in the

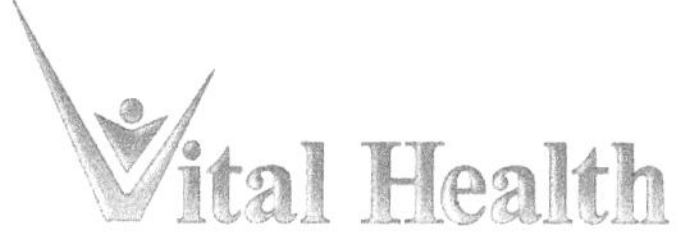

grocery stores. Farmed elk is light, lean and tender. It is rich in minerals like iron and phosphorous which is why the meat is dark in colour.[cxiii]

Comparative Nutritional Values Based on 100 Gram Meat Portions

	CALORIES	FAT (G)	CHOLESTEROL (MG)	PROTEIN(G)
Elk Meat, Loin Cut	159	3.3	56	25
Beef Bottom Round	214	9.7	692	31
Ground Beef	265	18.4	85	24
Pork Shoulder Cut	219	10.64	101	29
Lamb Leg Roast	178	7.62	83	25
Veal Cutlet	213	10.35	125	26
Chicken Breast	159	3.42	83	31
Turkey (light meat)	154	3.42	68	29
Salmon (pink)	138	5.75	39	20
Scallops (breaded)	215	11.0	77	17

Mineral Compositions MG Per 100 G Fresh Meat

	PHOSPHORUS	SODIUM	POTASSIUM	IRON	CALCIUM
Elk Meat, Loin	250	52	320	3.82	9.1
Beef Loin Steer	208	39	399	2.30	3.0
Beef Loin Heifer	210	40	417	2.20	2.9
Lamb Loin (castrated)	168	71	04	1.48	11.7
Lamb Loin Ram	167	77	314	1.40	13.7
Pork	200	76	370	.90	8.0
Chicken (white meat)	210	72	330	.50	10.0
Veal Cutlet	260	110	360	1.20	8.0

(Venison Consumption in the USA, (1992) Saskatchewan Agriculture and Food Department)

Kale

Kale is one of the most nutritious vegetables with only 36 calories per cup, which contains five grams of fibre. It's effective in aiding in digestion and elimination with its high fibre, vitamin, folate (Note. Vitamin B9 is naturally occurring in vegetables, fruits, grains, nuts, seeds, etc.[cxiv]) and magnesium content. It also has more iron than beef which is essential for the formation of hemoglobin, enzymes and transporting oxygen to the various systems of the body for cell growth, liver function, etc.[cxv]

Broccoli

Broccoli is a flower top vegetable that is picked before it blooms. It is dense in nutrition, full of beta carotene, high in fibre, high in vitamin B1, C, calcium, sulfur, and potassium. Forty-five percent of the calories are protein. The National Cancer Institute links a substance called inderol-3, which emulsifies estrogen, to reducing the risk of breast cancer in women.[cxvi]

EVENING SNACK

You can choose one of the following options as your evening snack:

- 1 cup herbal tea or 1 - 2 cup filtered water
- 8 - 14 oz of protein shake
- 6 - 10 whole grain organic crackers, brown rice crackers or Mary's Organic Crackers (Gluten Free) with the following toppings:
- 1 tbsp organic almond butter or tahini sauce
- 1 tsp apple butter or organic fruit jam
- 4 - 8oz fruits for evening snack (Note: you wait about 3 hours until you have fruit after supper so you don't experience fermentation in your digestive system)

Protein Utilization: How much is absorbed

Since I spent a significant amount of time as a bodybuilder in the gym trying to gain more muscle size and strength, the need to get enough protein was always on my mind. Dr. Franco Columbu, past pro-bodybuilder and Mr. Olympia winner, presents the following list of the best foods for protein and their protein absorption rates. As a bodybuilder or anyone trying to gain muscle size, you must consider the net protein utilization (NPU) or rate of protein absorption into the bloodstream. For those who are trying to lose weight, you need to be aware that some meat items are much higher in fat than others. For example, beef and chicken both have an absorption rate of 68 percent, yet chicken has the advantage of easier digestibility and contains almost half the calories of an equal weight of beef, pork or lamb. Hence, the reason why bodybuilders or people who are leaning up usually eat more chicken when trying to get more definition in their muscles.

The protein utilization rate of some common foods are as follows:

FOOD	NPU
Eggs	88%
Fish	78%
Dairy products	76%
Meat	68%
Soybeans	48%
Natural brown rice	40%
Red beans	39%
Coconut	38%
Nuts	35%
White beans	33%
Maize	25%
Whole wheat bread	21%
White bread	20%

The average person needs a daily intake of one gram of protein for every kilogram (2.2 pounds) of body weight. Adult males should consume 75-100 grams per day; however, an extra amount of protein is required to build muscular weight for those in heavy training. The food intake tables were calculated to accommodate both male and female bodybuilders and athletes whose goals range widely from training for good health and a vigorous appearance to entering competition at championship levels. My own intake of protein is high due to a schedule of weight training, circuit training and some recreational running, so I always try to choose the best sources. In addition to eating only prime cuts of meat and making a point of having fresh fish, I also include eggs in my daily food intake since they have the highest protein utilization rate, as noted above.

When the consumption of protein is increased, the body does not automatically secrete more hydrochloric acid (HCI) to aid digestion. Therefore, if you have significantly increased your intake of protein, it may be necessary to take HCI (hydrochloric acid) and digestive enzyme supplements to help digest the extra protein. I take extra probiotic supplements that have plant enzymes combined with good bacteria and drink a glass of fresh vegetable juice made in a juicer. I find the extra enzymes from the raw vegetables help digest the extra meat intake.

Be aware of the fat content of meats and various carbohydrate foods. Those having problems with excess weight should select items high in protein, but low in fat. For instance, there is little difference between the protein content of sirloin and round steaks, yet sirloin contains approximately 2.5 times more fat. Bear in mind that not all fat in meat is visible and that some cuts may contain over 40 percent fat, even if you have been very careful to trim off visible fat. Hamburgers sold in fast food chains have a notoriously high fat content, which may be the reason you feel more satisfied after eating one out than after eating one at home. Being more difficult to digest, fat remains in the stomach longer and gives a feeling of being full for an extended period of time.

Regarding foods from plant sources, keep in mind that only soybeans contain a significant amount of essential amino acids, but their balance is not the same as that found in meat, eggs, and fish. Since they have a limited amount of methionine, one of the essential amino acids your body needs, you have to consume a lot more of soybeans than meat to supply enough of the complete protein necessary for building muscle tissue. You probably noticed that fruit and vegetables are not listed with the protein foods. Many vegetable items contain less than three grams of protein, so they cannot be considered an efficient source of this nutrient.

"Many of the popular foods have been excluded from the protein foods list. Frozen breaded fish sticks, for example are not high-quality protein, no matter what the manufacturer has chosen to claim on their label. Fresh food in its most natural form always takes first place. Also, it is doubtful if an 8-ounce package of fish sticks actually contains 38 grams of protein from the fish itself. More likely, a high percentage of this amount comes from substances used for breading. The list is intended mainly to provide an awareness of protein sources.

In summary, the best bodybuilding foods from animal sources are fish, meat, eggs and poultry. Dairy products like cheese are high in protein, but also high in fat. Consuming cheese tends to form fat deposits under the skin, causing loss of definition. The best foods from plant sources are beans, nuts, seeds and grain products."

(By Dr. Franco Columbu, Mr Olympia past pro-bodybuilder, columbu.com)

About Sample Meal Programs

The meal plans on the following pages for females and males are designed for people who are not in a regular training program in the gym and who are not doing intense activities like running 10 Km and doing cross-fit classes three times a week. If you are doing these activities, then add another 600 calories worth of food to the plans.

The sample Female Lean Meal Program is for the average female adult who does not train intensely in a gym and who wants a meal plan that is healthy and balanced. With this plan, they should be able to maintain a fairly lean body composition, but not feel like they are on a strict calorie-reduced program. This is a high protein, moderate carb and fat meal plan. It has enough carb foods, but should not cause fat gain because much of the carb is coming from vegetable sources, whole grains and seeds, not from processed carb foods with refined sugars in them. Also, the fat portion of the meals is coming from organic meat choices and fish oil supplement. What makes this plan different from other meal plans out there is the many organic and whole food options.

The only real difference with the Athletic Female Meal Program is that the calories, protein and carbohydrate amounts are higher. It can even be higher than what is shown in the program sheets if the female athlete needs more food to fuel her training and sport needs. For example a female tri-athlete may need to consume double the amount of calories, carb and fat levels shown because the extreme amount of cardio training would demand it. Furthermore, the Male

Lean Meal Program also has a higher amounts of calories, protein, fat and carbohydrates because in most cases they carry a higher amount of body mass and greater level of muscle ratio. This would cause the male body to demand more calories since calorie and fat burning capacity of increased muscle ratio is higher. Again, if you are starting a training program at the gym at least three times a week I suggest you add another 600 calories to the Male Lean Meal Program.

The Male Mass Meal Program is for already serious males who are on an intense training program and are already quite developed. If you are a serious runner, tri-athlete, power lifter or bodybuilder, etc. then this meal program is for you. It is double the calories of the Male Lean Meal Program. It is for males who want to gain serious muscle size and more weight as well. The plan is an approximate calorie count of the food groups. You can easily go past that minimum to over 5,000 calories per day. I have personally gone past 5,000 to 6,000 calorie meal plans in the past to gain size. I was lifting heavy and training at least 3 - 4 times a week on top of my full time job which, was physically demanding as well. This meal plan is much higher in calories, protein and carb levels. If you are training for power-lifting, a bodybuilding show or training in the gym to make gains for your sport like football, soccer, rugby, etc., I suggest you make sure your calorie intake is 4,000 to 5,000 and your protein intake be between 200-300 grams. Your carb level should be around 250 grams minimum.

For this meal program, you can have some meals with protein and carbs together. The reason that I allow this is because you have to consume enough calories to gain size and there are not enough hours in a day to fit in all the meals if you separated the carbs and protein. What I also recommend is that you take extra digestive enzymes and probiotic supplements to help digest the high level of protein that your body has to breakdown. Furthermore, I suggest you also have extra raw vegetable juices done in the juice machine fresh every day, which will also help to digest the extra amount of protein, fats and carbs you are consuming.

I also suggest you use some glutamine for recovery of the sore muscles and for better digestion. I add about two four-gram scoops of glutamine into my protein shake each day. Over 60 percent of skeletal muscle is made up of glutamine. It is also good for structural intestinal health.

I recommend adding about three four-gram scoops of BCAAs (Branch Chain Amino Acids) to your shake every day as well. This helps on a molecular level to gain muscle, but keeps you from losing too much muscle when leaning down for a bodybuilding or physique show. The challenge of bodybuilding is to try to stay lean while at the same time try to gain size. When on a strict diet to get lean while training hard, the body tries hard to hold onto fat stores. In the process, the body will use up muscle for its energy needs, hence muscle breakdown and loss of size occurs.

Another supplement I add to my shake is creatine. I usually add about a 4 - 6 gram scoops to my shake every day. Creatine is a protein-like compound found in high abundance in meat and fish. It is synthesized in the body, primarily in the liver from three amino acids; arginine, glycine and methionine. Muscle cells get creatine from the bloodstream. In the muscle cells creatine gets a high-energy phosphate attached to it and then it is known as phosphocreatine (PCr) or creatine phosphate. This is a high energy molecule because it donates its phosphate to create ATP, which is the energy molecule that causes the muscle to contract. Therefore, taking extra creatine means increased (PCr) in the muscle by 20 percent that translates to increased energy which leads to gains in strength, power, speed, and muscle growth. Although there is some controversy over the use of creatine, there is much more research showing positive benefits for people who want to make gains in their overall training goals. I personally have experienced the difference it makes in my performance in the gym and in other sports activities.

Along with all the previous supplements mentioned, I also recommend a good quality non-flavoured or naturally flavoured whey isolate to combine with the fruit to make your protein shake. When you are trying to gain muscle size and strength, you need high amounts of protein. I then add a third of a pack of the vegetarian meal replacement Pure Trim to my mix. This not only makes it taste better, but adds in all the other food nutrients like omega oils, herbal extracts, vegetables, algae, etc., turning the shake into a total meal. A final natural ingredient I use is Maca powder, known to increase the fertility in men and women and which has hormone balancing effects on the body. Maca boosts the energy level, but unlike coffee it does not stress the adrenals. Its energy level effect is even and sustained.

I personally use it in my shakes almost every day and I notice a difference in my strength and stamina in the gym.

STRENGTH AND MASS PROTEIN SHAKE RECIPE:

- 2 1/2 cups of filtered water
- 1 ripe banana
- 4 - 6 oz of fresh fruit or frozen
- 2 heaping scoops of whey isolate protein powder
- 1/3 pack of chocolate vegetarian Pure Trim shake
- 3 level scoops of BCAAs
- 2 level 30 g scoops creatine monohydrate
- 2 level 30 g scoops glutamine
- 1 level tsp of Maca powder

When you are training for a bodybuilding show the amount of training can be three to four hours per day, four to five times a week. The amount of energy output is high, so you have to keep track and make sure you are staying ahead of the catabolism that can occur from all the training. Make sure you consume enough protein to maintain size and enough carbs to have enough energy to have effective workouts. In addition, these meals have a high amount of nutrients, combined with raw vegetables that have lots of micronutrients which help keep the immune system high and help with recovery after training. If you are training and also keeping up with team practices, you have a challenge. Especially in sports like football and soccer where there is explosive sprinting where the cardio fat burn can be quite high. I would suggest increasing carb levels to over 250 grams and even over 300 grams.

I have underlined the importance of the calorie amount as something to be aware of, but the nutrient density of your food is just as important. For instance, a processed snack bar that is 100 calories is still not as good as a large apple of about the same caloric amount. For instance, an apple has Vitamin C, folate, fibre, potassium, Vitamin B6, thiamin, and riboflavin. The nutrient value of the apple would be a lot higher than the snack bar which may also have three to four different kinds of sugars.

As we age, another challenge we face is a drop in testosterone which affects weight-loss, strength, motivation, fat-burning, skin tone, bone density, libido, memory and muscle gain. Being able to maintain a healthy level of testosterone is what allows us to still have vigor, high energy and strength for an active lifestyle as we age. It helps keep us "young" to a certain degree. If you are severely low, then there is a testosterone cream you can get through your Medical Doctor (MD) or Naturopathc Doctor (ND). In the Supplement section, there are some additional natural supplements that can be used to increase testosterone levels.

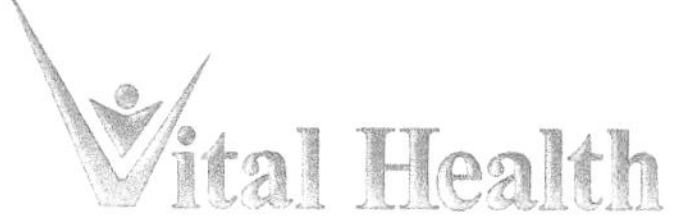

FEMALE LEAN MEAL PLAN

UPON WAKING	CAL.	PROTEIN(G)	FAT(G)	CARB(G)
Drink 3 to 6 glasses of water upon the first hour and half of waking up (Note. 8 glasses of water if wrong combination of foods eaten the day before)				
Bowl of fresh fruit with sprinkle of cinnamon (Note. 4-8 oz banana, apples, nectarines, berries, etc.)	50	0.5	Tr	26
(Note. wait half hour to digest the fruit as you drink the water before breakfast) 1 tbsp omega-3 oil or 3 capsules of fish oil, one powder capsule 50 mg. Vitamin B complex, 1 level tsp Vitamin C powder (about 1500 mg) 2 level tbsp of liquid Daily Complete	130	0	13.5	0
BREAKFAST A (Note. you have the option of only having breakfast A or B in the mornings, hence your calorie total for the day will be less; however you can have both on days you are hungry)				
(Note. I suggest not to use milk, but if you really find it hard to change, please use organic milk)				
4-8 oz organic milk, almond, rice milk, or goat's milk	45	4.5		6
4 oz organic oatmeal, quinoa, millet, or seed cereal	65	1	1	11.5
8-12 oz veg. / fruit juice from juice machine (Note. 4-6 carrots, celery, chunk of beet, apple and 1 inch chunk ginger root)	69	1.9	0.35	16.1
BREAKFAST B 12 oz of garden salad or sliced cucumbers, tomatoes, green pepper, celery, carrots, zucchini, etc. & 1 tbsp vinaigrette	50	3	0	7
1 egg (Note. free range egg, poached, boiled or scrambled) & 1 cup herbal tea	80	6	6	
MID-MORNING SNACK (OPTIONAL IF HUNGRY) 1 c of protein shake (Note. whey isolate, Pure Trim or both)	86	14.6	1.3	4
(Note. Recipe for 3 cup protein shake: 2.5 cups of water, 1 banana, 4 oz. fresh or frozen strawberries, ½ pack Pure Trim shake and 2 scoops unflavoured whey isolate)				

LUNCH (Note. drink 1.5 to 2 cups of water)				
4 oz organic chicken, turkey, free range beef, lamb, or wild fish (Note. marinate with spices, garlic)	309	30.6	20	0
8-12 oz broccoli, Brussell sprouts, green beans, kale, cauliflower, etc., with a ½ tsp of sea salt and ground pepper	40	4.5	0.5	7.5
8-12 oz salad, 1 tsp organic salad dressing	67	0	6.5	7
MID-NOON SNACK Drink 1.5 to 2 cups of water before meal				
4-8 oz pineapple or other fruits (Note. wait half hour before having protein snack)	50	.5		26
½ oz of almonds, walnuts or pecans	78	2.4	6.3	4.1
SUPPER (Note. drink 1.5 to 2 cups of water)				
8 oz organic soup, i.e. squash or roasted pepper tomato soup	72	2	2	12
4 oz chicken, beef, lamb, seafood or wild fish	309	30.6	20	0
16 oz non-starch vegetables like broccoli, spinach, carrots, kale, Swiss chard, turnip, spinach, asparagus, green beans etc.	30	2	0	7
12 oz Salad 1 tbsp vinaigrette dressing	50	3	0	7
oz low sugar fruits (Note. i.e. bananas, pears, oranges, grapes, etc.) & 1 cup herbal tea (optional)	20	0.3	Tr	4.6
TOTALS:	**1580**	**107.1**	**77.5**	**141.2**

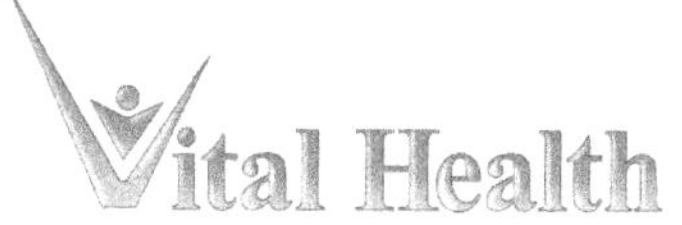

ATHLETIC FEMALE LEAN MEAL PLAN

UPON WAKING	CAL.	PROTEIN(G)	FAT(G)	CARB(G)
Drink 3 to 6 glasses of water upon the first hour and half of waking up (Note. 8 glasses of water if wrong combination of foods were eaten the day before)				
Bowl of fresh fruit with sprinkle of cinnamon, 4-8 oz banana, apples, nectarines, berries, etc., wait half hour to digest before breakfast	50	0.5	Tr	26
BREAKFAST A (Note. you have the option of only having breakfast A or B in the mornings, hence your calorie total for the day will be less; however you can have both on days you are hungry)				
4-6 oz goat's milk, home-made almond milk, unsweetened store almond milk or rice milk (Note. if you really find it hard to change, please at least get organic milk)	45	4.5	Tr	6
4 oz organic oatmeal, quinoa, millet or seed cereal (Note. have the seed cereal every other day and have one of the other cereals like oatmeal, quinoa or millet)	65	1	1	11.5
8-12 oz veg. / fruit juice from juice machine (Note. 4-6 carrots, celery, chunk of beet, apple and 1 inch chunk ginger root)	69	1.9	0.35	16.1
BREAKFAST B 8 - 12 oz Salad 1 tbsp vinaigrette	50	3	0	7
2 free range eggs or 4 oz seafood, chicken, turkey, tuna	160	12	12	0
1 tbsp omega-3 oil or 3 capsules of fish oil, one powder capsule 50 mg vitamin B complex, 1 level tsp Vitamin C powder (about 1500 mg),				
2 level tbsp of liquid Daily Complete	130	0	13.5	0
1 cup herbal tea				
LUNCH (Note. drink 1.5 to 2 cups of water)				
4 oz lean chicken, beef, turkey, or seafood	186	22.5	6	.5
8 oz potato, yam, squash, brown rice,	332	4	Tr	77.2
16 oz broccoli, cauliflower, green beans, etc.	160	18	2	30
or 12 oz salad 1 tbsp vinaigrette or oil & balsamic or organic salad dressing	249	5	22	10.7

MID-NOON SNACK (Note. drink 1.5 to 2 cups of water)				
1 c of protein shake				
(Note. Recipe for 3 cup protein shake: 2.5 cups of water, 1 or ½ banana, 4 - 6 oz fresh fruit or frozen fruit, ½ pack Pure Trim shake or unflavoured whey isolate)	86	15	1.3	4
4 oz fruits with 4 oz organic plain yogurt	185	6	2	18
SUPPER (Note. drink 1.5 to 2 cups of water)				
4 oz fish/ chicken, turkey, seafood, or meat stew,	186	22.5	6	.5
16-20 oz non-starch vegetables like broccoli, spinach, carrots, kale, Swiss chard, turnip, spinach, asparagus, green beans etc.	30	2	0	7
12-16 oz salad with 1 tbsp organic salad dressing	167	9	6.5	21
1 tbsp omega-3 oil or 2 capsules of fish oil	32	0	13.5	0
EVENING SNACK 4-6 organic gluten free grain crackers	65	1.6	1.7	11
1 tbsp organic almond butter	95	4	8	3
1 tbsp apple butter or organic jams sweetened with grape juice or raw sugar	55	Tr	Tr	14
TOTALS:	**1828**	**109.6**	**69.0**	**196.9**

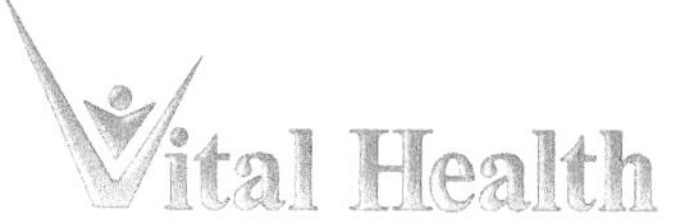

MALE LEAN MEAL PLAN

UPON WAKING	CAL.	PROTEIN(G)	FAT(G)	CARB(G)
Drink 3 to 6 glasses of water upon the first hour and half of waking up (Note. 8 glasses of water if wrong combination of foods eaten the day before)				
Bowl of fresh fruit with sprinkle of cinnamon (Note. 4 - 8 oz fruits i.e. banana, apple, nectarine, berries, etc.)	50	0.5	Tr	26
(Note. wait half hour to digest the fruit before breakfast)				
BREAKFAST A (Note. you have the option of only having breakfast A or B in the mornings, hence your calorie total for the day will be less; however you can have both on days you are hungry)				
6-8 oz almond, goat's milk, or rice milk	45	4.5	Tr	6
4-8 oz organic oatmeal, quinoa, millet or seed cereal every other day (Note. have the other cereals on the other days)	65	1	1	11.5
8-12 oz veg. / fruit juice from juice machine (Note. 4-6 carrots, celery, chunk of beet, apple and 1 inch chunk ginger root)	69	1.9	0.35	16.1
BREAKFAST B 8 - 12 oz salad and 1 tbsp vinaigrette	50	3	0	7
2 free range eggs or 4 oz seafood, chicken, turkey, tuna	160	12	12	0
1 tbsp omega-3 or 2 capsules of omega-3 fish oil, one powder capsule 50 mg vitamin B complex, 1 level tsp Vitamin C powder (about 1500 mg),				
2 level tbsp of liquid Daily Complete	130	0	13.5	0
1 cup herbal tea (Note. add ½ tsp honey optional)				
LUNCH (Note. drink 1.5 to 2 cups of water)				
4 oz lean organic chicken, free range beef, lamb, turkey, wild fish or seafood	186	22.5	6	.5
16 oz broccoli, cauliflower, green beans, or kale, etc.	160	18	2	30
12 oz salad with 1 tbsp vinaigrette dressing	50	3	0	7

MID-NOON SNACK (Note. total calorie of the day includes all the snacks, therefore when you only have one of the snacks the total calorie will be less)				
4 oz pineapple, fruit with	41			10
4 oz organic low fat plain yogurt	72	6	2	8
or 12 oz green vegetable smoothie	204	2.1	6.5	21.4
(Note. Smoothie Recipe: 3 cups water, 2 cups organic spinach, 1 apple, 1 pear cored and chopped, half an avocado and 1-2 inch chunk ginger)				
SUPPER (Note. drink 1.5 to 2 cups of water)				
8 oz wild fish, organic chicken, or turkey	186	22.5	6	.5
16 oz non-starch vegetables like broccoli, spinach, carrots, kale, Swiss chard, turnip, spinach, asparagus, or green beans etc.	160	18	2	30
12 oz salad with 1 tbsp vinaigrette	50	3	0	7
4 oz low sugar fruits for desert	20			4.6
EVENING SNACK 1 c of protein shake				
(Note. Recipe for 3 cup protein shake: 2.5 cups of water, 1 or ½ banana, 4-6 oz fresh fruit or frozen fruit, ½ pack Pure Trim shake or unflavoured whey isolate	86	15	1.3	4
1 cup herbal tea	0	0	0	0
TOTALS:	**1784**	**133**	**52.65**	**189.6**

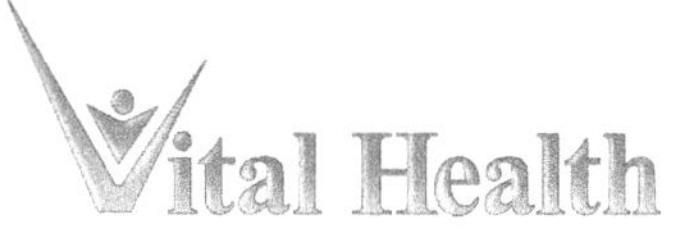

MALE MASS MEAL PLAN

UPON WAKING	CAL.	PROTEIN (G)	FAT (G)	CARB (G)
Drink 3 to 6 glasses of water upon the first hour and half of waking up (Note. 8 glasses of water if wrong combination of foods eaten the day before)				
Bowl of fresh fruit with sprinkle of cinnamon (4-8 oz fruits i.e., banana, apple, nectarine, berries, etc.)	50	0.5	Tr	26
(Wait half hour to digest the fruit as you drink the water before breakfast)				
BREAKFAST A (Note. you have the option of only having breakfast A or B in the mornings, hence your calorie total for the day will be less; however you can have both on days you are hungry)				
4 oz goat's milk, almond milk, or rice milk				
4 oz organic oatmeal, quinoa, millet or seed cereal				
(Note. have the seed cereal every other day and have one of the other cereals like oatmeal, quinoa or millet)	65	1	1	11.5
8 oz vegetable juice from juice machine (Note. 4-6 carrots, celery, chunk of beet, apple and 1 inch chunk ginger root)	69	1.9	0.35	16.1
BREAKFAST B 12 oz salad with 1 tbsp of oil & balsamic or organic salad dressing	167	9	6.5	21
3-43 - 4 eggs & 8 oz organic beef steak or ground lean beef (Note. free range eggs and grass fed beef)	533	70	32	0
12 oz glass of protein shake				
(Note. Recipe of protein shake: 2.5 cups of water, 1 banana, 4-6 oz fresh fruit or frozen fruit, ½ pack Pure Trim shake and 2 heaping scoops of unflavoured whey isolate, 4-6 gram scoop of creatine, three 4 gram scoop of BCAA, two 4 gram scoop of glutamine and a level tsp of Maca powder)	160	27.5	0.65	14.7
1 tbsp omega-3 or 3 capsules omega-3 fish oil, one powder capsule 50 mg vitamin B complex, 1 level tsp Vitamin C powder (about 1500 mg), 2 level tbsp of liquid Daily Complete	130	0	13.5	0

MID-MORNING SNACK 1 slice organic kamut, spelt bread, 8 oz yam, or potato	175	2	1.3	40
1 tbsp organic almond butter	95	4	8	3
8 oz green smoothie (Note. smoothie Recipe: 3 cups water, 2 cups organic spinach, 1 apple, 1 pear cored and chopped, half an avocado and 1-2 inch chunk ginger)	214	6	20	
LUNCH (Note. drink 1.5 to 2 cups of water)				
12 oz glass of protein shake	160	27.5	0.65	14.7
8-12 oz organic chicken, fish, or beef	306.2	53	7.8	0
1 cup herbal tea				
1 tbsp omega-3 or 3 capsules omega-3 fish oil	130	0	13.5	0
8 oz steamed vegetables	30	2	0	7
8 oz potato, yam, squash, or brown rice	205	5.2	0.4	20.5
MID-NOON SNACK 4 oz seed cereal, oatmeal, or granola	130	2	2	23
12 oz glass of protein shake	160	27.5	0.65	14.7
4 oz green beans or non-starch vegetables	15	1	0	3.5
8 oz skinless organic chicken, baked, broiled or barbeque	306.2	53	7.8	0
SUPPER (Note. drink 1.5 to 2 cups of water)				
1 cup protein shake	160	27.5	0.65	14.7
8-12 oz organic chicken, fish, or beef	448	12	12	0
12 oz green beans, broccoli, spinach, carrots, kale, Swiss chard, turnip, spinach, asparagus, etc.	160	18	2	30
8 oz potato, yam, squash, or brown rice	205	5.2	0.4	20.5
12 oz salad with 1 tbsp organic salad dressing	214	6	20	
EVENING SNACK 12 oz glass protein shake & glass of water (optional 1 cup of herbal tea)	160	27.5	0.65	2.5
1 tbsp omega-3 or 3 omega-3 capsules fish oil	130	0	13.5	0
TOTALS:	**4577.4**	**389.3**	**165.3**	**283.4**

Travelling and Eating

It is not always easy to find whole and organic foods when you are travelling. Here is a sample meal plan I have used for clients who travel frequently for their work.

TRAVEL MEAL PLAN

UPON WAKING	CAL.	PROTEIN(G)	FAT(G)	CARB(G)
Drink 3 to 6 glasses of water upon the first hour and half of waking up (Note. 8 glasses of water if wrong combination of foods eaten the day before)				
8 oz fruits i.e. banana, apple, nectarine, berries, etc. (Note. wait half hour to digest the fruit before breakfast)	50	0.5	Tr	26
BREAKFAST A (Note. you have the option of only having breakfast A or B in the mornings, hence your calorie total for the day will be less; however you can have both on days you are hungry)				
6-8 oz unsweetened almond milk, rice milk ,goat's milk or organic milk (Note. you can get these at a local health food store or large grocery store, if not, use 2% or skim milk as a last resort)	45	4.5	Tr	6

4-8 oz organic oatmeal, grain cereals or seed cereal (Note. you can find these cereals at a local health food store if there are no organic places or grind seed mixture cereal and carry it in zip lock bag)	65	1	1	11.5
BREAKFAST B 12 oz salad of lettuce, cucumber, tomato and celery with 1 tbsp vinaigrette	50	3	0	7
Scrambled eggs	160	12	12	0
3 capsules omega-3 fish oil, one powder capsule 50 mg vitamin B complex, 1 level tsp Vitamin C powder (about 1500 mg), 2 level tbsp of liquid Daily Complete	130	0	13.5	0
1 cup herbal tea				
LUNCH (Note. drink 1.5 to 2 cups of water)				
8 oz lean chicken, beef, turkey, or seafood	186.5	22.5	6	.5
8 oz potato, squash, brown rice, or whole wheat pasta	332	4	Tr	77.2
16 oz broccoli, cauliflower, carrots, green beans, etc.	160	18	2	30
16 oz salad 1 tbsp vinaigrette or olive oil and balsamic	249	5	22	10.7
MID-NOON SNACK 1 c of Pure Trim shake (Note. you can empty half pack of pure trim in 8 oz water and shake in a bottle)	86	15	1.3	4
Or 1 oz raw cashews, almonds	157	4.8	12.8	8.2
SUPPER (Note. drink 1.5 to 2 cups of water)				
4 oz beef, fish, chicken, turkey, or seafood	186.5	22.5	6	.5
12 oz non-starch vegetables like broccoli, spinach, carrots, kale, Swiss chard, turnip, spinach, asparagus, green beans etc.	30	2	0	7
12 oz salad 1 tbsp vinaigrette	50	3	0	7
EVENING SNACK 8 oz fruits i.e. banana, apple, nectarine, berries, etc.	50	0.5	Tr	26
1 cup herbal tea	0	0	0	0
TOTALS:	**1987**	**118.3**	**76.6**	**221.6**

Foods for Health Conditions

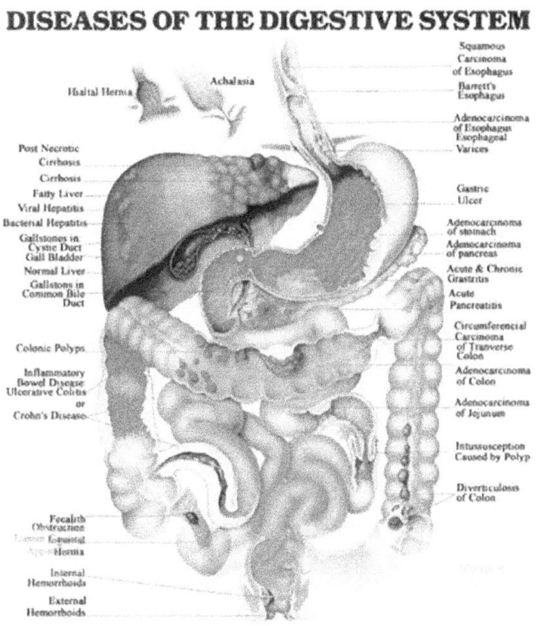

FOODS FOR HEALTH ISSUES

People may struggle with common ailments due to poor diet and lifestyle, genetic disposition, or from the result of trauma. It may not be possible to entirely reverse a health condition, but these meal and supplement plans will make a significant difference in alleviating symptoms and increasing energy levels. Digestion, absorption and recovery will be greatly enhanced.

ANEMIA MEAL PLAN EXPLAINED

This meal plan contains twice the recommended amount of iron needed for adult males and females. Based on your body mass and your activity level, the portion size of each meal, snacks and protein shake can vary, but if you stay at least to even half of what is recommended in this meal chart, you will get enough iron. I also have the breakfast in two parts, A and B, for people who cannot eat both meals. Choose either one for breakfast. If you work out and are active, you may need to eat both A and B.

Recommended amounts of iron for adults per day:

- Women ages from 19-50, 18 mg
- Pregnant women ages 14-50, 27 mg
- Lactating women ages 14-19, 10 mg
- Lactating women ages 19-50, 9 mg
- Men ages 19-50, 8 mg
- Everyone over 51, 8 mg

DIABETIC MEAL PLAN EXPLAINED

Fruits: Try to eat fruits raw, no sugar added. A piece of fruit is preferable to juice as whole fruit is more filling and has more fibre. Save high sugar and fat desserts, such as apple pie, for special occasions only. If you buy from an organic bakery or restaurant, you can opt for desserts made from whole grains and sweetened with raw sugar, honey or maple syrup which, does not increase sugar levels as much as refined sugars.

Serving sizes for fruits:

- One serving can be one small apple or ½ cup of juice or ½ a grapefruit.
- Two servings can be one banana or ½ cup of unsweetened juice with 1 cup of apples.

Vegetables: Try to eat vegetables raw and steamed with little sauces, no fat or dressings. Use chicken broth made from soup base with no MSG. Add whatever spices you would like. Additions like garlic, lemon, or lime juice can be used. A teaspoon of cold-pressed olive oil can also be used.

Serving sizes for vegetables:

- 1 serving can be ½ cup of greens or a cup of salad
- 2 servings can be ½ cup of turnips with 1 cup of salad or ½ cup of fresh vegetable juice with ½ cup green beans
- 3 servings can be ½ cup of peas with ½ cup of carrots and 1 small tomato or ½ cup broccoli with 1 cup of zucchini

Starches: Organic whole grains, sprouted grain breads, whole grain pastas, tortilla, sweet potato, white potato, wild rice and brown rice are the best choices. Use low fat organic sour cream – if you must – on potatoes. Use only about a half teaspoon of organic mayonnaise or mustard on a sandwich. Stick to organic cereals sweetened with honey, no preservatives. Organic steel-cut oats, millet, granola and quinoa are good choices.

Serving sizes for starches:

- 1 serving can be 1 slice of organic bread or 1 small potato or ½ cup of organic granola
- 2 servings can be 1 small potato with half cob of corn or 2 slices of organic bread
- 3 servings can be 1 slice organic bread, ½ cup of green beans and 1 small potato or 1 cup of brown rice

Protein: Stick to lean cuts of meat with all fat trimmed. Eat chicken and turkey skinless. Cook meats in low-fat methods like broiling, grill, roast, steam and BBQ. Use wine, lemon juice, balsamic vinegars, low sodium tamari sauce, herbs and spices on meats instead of rich sauces. Use an olive-oil spray when cooking eggs or meat on the pan. Keep consumption of nut butters to a minimum and stay away from fried foods. Eat cheeses sparingly (i.e. 30 g slice once a week) and opt for low fat. Get organic free-range meats as much as possible because they are not only hormone free and preservative free, but also leaner.

Serving sizes for meats:
- 1 serving is 3-4 oz
- 2 servings is 6-8 oz

Examples of fat foods:
- Organic Salad dressing
- Butter
- Avocado
- Olives
- Ricotta cheese
- Cheeses
- Organic Mayonnaise
- Organic Turkey Bacon

Examples of sweets:
- Organic Cake
- Organic Pie
- Organic Cookies
- Soya Ice cream
- Pure Maple Syrup

Examples of 1 serving of sweets:
- One three inch organic cookie
- One organic muffin
- One tbsp pure maple syrup

In the Diabetic Meal Plan, I have given some options for evening snacks; therefore the total calorie count is actually probably less than 1900. I included all three evening snack options to the total calories for the day.

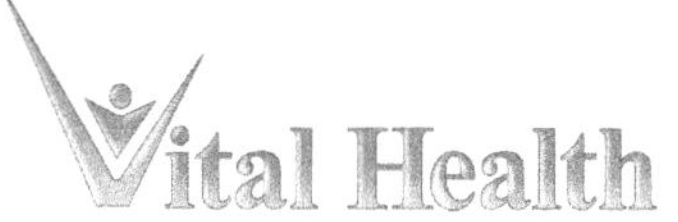

ANEMIA MEAL PLAN

UPON WAKING	CAL.	PROTEIN(G)	FAT(G)	CARB(G)
Drink 3 to 7 glasses of water upon the first hour and half of waking up (Note. 8 glasses of water if wrong combination of foods eaten the day before)				
Bowl of fresh fruit with sprinkle of cinnamon (Note. 4-8 oz banana, apples, nectarines, berries, etc.)				
Add 1 tbsp of raisins	77	0.7	0	33
(Note. Wait half hour to digest the fruit before breakfast)				
1 tbsp omega-3 oil or 3 capsules of fish oil, one powder capsule 50 mg vitamin B complex, 1 level tsp Vitamin C powder (about 1500 mg)				
2 level tbsp of liquid Daily Complete	130	0	13.5	0
BREAKFAST A (Note. you have the option of only having breakfast A or B in the mornings, hence your calorie total for the day will be less; however you can have both on days you are hungry)				
(Note. I suggest not to use milk with cereal but if you really find it hard to change, please at least get organic milk)				
8 oz. organic almond milk (about .7 mg iron per cup)	45	4.5		6
4 oz. organic oatmeal (about 14mg iron)	77	2.5	1.5	13.5
8-12 oz veg. / fruit Juice (4 oz. spinach, about 6 carrots and apple gives about 1.5 mg iron)	69	1.9	0.35	16.1
BREAKFAST B 12 oz garden salad of sliced cucumbers, tomatoes, green pepper, celery and 4 oz. spinach & 1 tbsp vinaigrette (1.3 mg iron) & 1 cup herbal tea	50	3	0	7
2 free range eggs (boiled or scrambled, 1.4 mg iron)	160	12	10	1
Mid-morning snack (optional if hungry)				
1 c of protein shake (has approx. 1.2 mg iron)	86	14.6	1.3	4
(Note. Recipe for 3 cup protein shake: 2.5 cups of water, 1 banana, 4 oz. fresh or frozen strawberries, ½ pack Pure Trim shake and 2 scoops unflavoured whey isolate)				

LUNCH (Note. drink 1.5 to 2 cups of water)				
4 oz. beef, lamb, chicken giblets, turkey giblets, or beef liver (meal can have 3mg to 7mg of iron)	309	31	20	0
8 oz. broccoli, Brussell sprouts, green beans, kale, or cauliflower, etc., with a ½ tsp of sea salt, ground pepper (.9 mg iron)	40	4.5	0.5	7.5
12 oz. salad with 1 tbsp oil & balsamic or lemon juice and organic salad dressing (1.3 mg iron)	249	5	22	10.7
MID-NOON SNACK (Note. drink 1.5 to 2 cups of water)				
4 oz. low fat organic yogurt with 1 tbsp almonds (1 mg iron)	124	8	6.5	10
SUPPER (Note. drink 1.5 to 2 cups of water)				
8 oz. organic soup, i.e. squash or tomato soup	72	2	2	12
4 oz. beef, lamb, chicken giblets, turkey giblets, or beef liver (meal can have 3mg to 7mg of iron)	309	31	20	0
8 oz. broccoli, Brussell sprouts, green beans, kale, etc., ½ tsp of sea salt, ground pepper (.9 mg iron)	40	4.5	0.5	7.5
12 oz. salad with 1 tsp organic salad dressing (1.3 mg iron)	67	0	6.5	7
EVENING SNACK (Note. drink 1.5 to 2 cups of water)				
4 oz. fresh fruits (Note. wait 30 minutes then eat the snack) & 1 cup herbal tea	20	0.3	Tr	4.6
4-6 five grain, organic crackers or rice crackers				
1 tbsp organic almond butter (1.2 mg iron)	203	4	14	21
TOTALS:	**2127**	**129.5**	**118.65**	**160.9**

DIABETIC MEAL PLAN

UPON WAKING	CAL.	PROTEIN(G)	FAT(G)	CARBS (G)
Drink 3 to 6 glasses of water upon the first hour and half of waking up (Note. 8 glasses of water if wrong combination of foods eaten the day before)				
2 servings of fresh fruit with sprinkle of cinnamon, i.e.1 banana or 1 cup of fruit mixture of your choice.	105	1	Tr	27
(Note. wait half hour to digest the fruit before breakfast)				
1 tbsp omega-3 oil or 3 capsules of fish oil, one powder capsule 50 mg vitamin B complex, 1 level tsp Vitamin C powder (about 1500 mg)				
2 level tbsp of liquid Daily Complete	130	0	13.5	0
BREAKFAST A (Note. you have the option of only having breakfast A or B in the mornings, hence your calorie total for the day will be less; however you can have both on days you are hungry)				
(Note. I suggest not to use milk with cereal but if you really find it hard to change, please at least get organic milk)				
8 oz organic 2% milk, almond, rice milk, or goats milk	45	4.5		6
4 oz organic oatmeal, quinoa, millet, or seed cereal	65	1	1	11.5
4 oz veg. juice (Note. made fresh in juice machine)	69	1.9	0.35	16.1
BREAKFAST B 8 oz salad 1 tbsp oil & balsamic, lemon juice or				
organic salad dressing	67	0	6.5	7
1 tbsp vinaigrette or olive oil & balsamic dressing, apple cider vinegar or squeezed lemon juice	119		14	
1-2 free range eggs (poached, boiled or scrambled)	160	12	12	0
1 cup herbal tea				
LUNCH (Note. drink 1.5 to 2 cups of water)				
4 oz skinless chicken or turkey roasted, broiled, etc.				
(with spices and garlic)	186	34	4	0
8 oz broccoli, Brussell sprouts, green beans, kale, cauliflower, etc., ½ tsp of sea salt, ground pepper	40	4.5	0.5	7.5

MID-NOON SNACK (Note. drink 1.5 to 2 cups of water)				
4 oz berries (Note. wait 30 minutes then eat carb meal)	109			27
4 oz potato/yam, squash, brown rice, whole wheat pasta, vermicelli noodles or Japanese soba noodles	166	2	Tr	38.5
SUPPER (Note. drink 1.5 to 2 cups of water)				
4 oz organic soup, i.e. squash or tomato soup	36	1	1	6
4 oz beef or lamb	309	31	20	0
8 oz non-starch vegetables like broccoli, spinach, carrots, kale, Swiss chard, turnip, spinach, asparagus, green beans etc.	15	1	Tr	3.5
12 oz salad 1 tbsp oil & balsamic, lemon juice or organic salad dressing	249	5	22	10.7
EVENING SNACK (Note. drink 1.5 to 2 cups of water)				
1 cup herbal tea & 4-6 five grain, organic crackers or rice crackers	65	1.6	1.7	11
1 tbsp organic almond or peanut butter OR	95	4	8	3
1 c of Pure Trim shake				
(Note. Recipe for 3 cup protein shake: 2.5 cups of water, 1 or ½ banana, 4-6 oz fresh fruit or frozen fruit, ½ pack Pure Trim shake or unflavoured whey isolate)	86	14.6	1.3	4
TOTALS:	**1934**	**114.1**	**90.35**	**175.1**

Overcoming Cancer

In the West, as well as in many other areas of the world, cancer has become the main health challenge and statistics confirm this. Two in every five people will experience cancer at some point in their life and only about half will survive five years from their diagnosis date. Even with all the advanced methods of surgery, radiotherapy and chemotherapy, usually the survival rate does not go past 25 percent. After a detailed analysis of the main causes of cancer, two-thirds are linked to lifestyle choices. It can be prevented. Just giving up smoking prevents it by 30 percent. Another 30 percent is linked to poor diet – a lack of enough fruits and vegetables.

Here is a short list based on research showing the direct impact of the various items that are linked to cancer:

Smoking – 30%
Diet – 30%
UV – 2%
Pollution – 2%
Infection – 5%
Obesity and lack of exercise – 5%
Workplace exposure – 5%
Drugs and alcohol – 5%

Cancer grows from precancerous cells which are cells that have mutated because of carcinogenic substances in the body, viruses, radiation or free radicals. They can also be acquired in the genes. They have the potential to become cancerous but will stay hidden and dormant as long as the cellular environment in which they live is not favourable for them to grow. For it to grow, it must avoid the surveillance of the immune system, and acquire a blood vessel network that will supply it with nutrients and oxygen. It must learn to reproduce itself without external help. Only when the precancerous cells mutate many times, does cancer gain strength to grow and invade the surrounding tissue in the body. In many cases, in a healthy body with a high immune system, there are only micro-tumours made up of several hundred thousands of cells. These are harmless and undetectable. It's only when a precancerous tumour grows to a volume of 1 cubic millimeter that it can be detected. Then it becomes dangerous and can invade the tissue quickly.

One of the best ways to fight and prevent precancerous cell growth is to make sure we consume enough foods of plant origin that contain phytochemical compounds that block precancerous cells from reaching their maturation. Another factor in the survival and growth of precancerous cells is the immune system cells that cause chronic inflammation which allows precancerous cells a blood vessel network for their energy needs. One of the best ways to prevent this is to have a diet abundant in plant origin with high amount of omega-3 fatty acids, which reduce inflammation of the cells. Salmon, mackerel, sardines and herring are full of omega-3. Include these fish as one of the main sources of protein in your regular meals. Another cause of cancer is obesity – too much food rich in calories, highly processed fods, and little physical activity. The increase in the adipose (fatty) tissue mass not only affects various body functions negatively, but it supports a pro-inflammatory environment that will help develop several types of cancers.

The best attack is through making the best lifestyle choices that will eliminate or greatly decrease the various causes of cancer, as shown on the previous list. From a nutritional approach, you can practice doing various cleanses to rid the body of toxins. You can follow the food plans as shown in this book. You can also spend regular time to perform 30 minutes of exercises using weights, your own body weight and accessories. Then you can add 30-45 minutes of some sort of cardio activity like walking, running, swimming, cross country skiing, etc. These lifestyle choices when practiced on a regular basis will greatly help to reduce excess

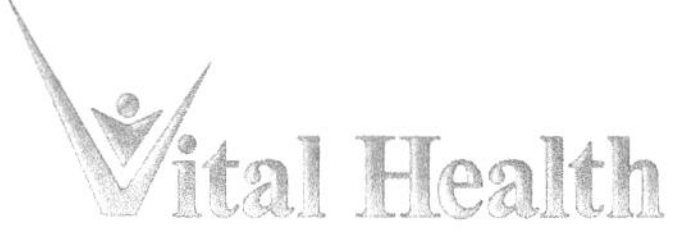

fat and maintain your body weight at a healthy level. If you smoke, you should make use of all the resources out there to quit. Also, eliminate regular alcohol consumption, use of recreational drugs and decrease as much as possible dependence on prescription drugs. Just by doing these five things you are preventing the growth of the precancerous cells by over 70 percent. Also, if you live in a country where the pollution factor is minimal and if you work in a more environmentally friendly work place where there are fewer chemicals, fumes, and electromagnetic waves, you increase your prevention percentage even more.

In the anti-cancer meal plan, you may want to change the various portion sizes of each meal according to how hungry you are and how much you need to eat to fuel your body. If you are physically active – running, swimming or exercising at the gym – you may need to increase the portion size of some of the meals. If you find the plan has too much food, cut down on the portion size of the meat and vegetables and cut out the snacks. What is important is sticking to eating the various food groups given.

Anti-Cancer Foods

POWER OF BERRIES

Berries such as strawberries and raspberries have a compound called Ellagic acid, and blueberries have anthocyanidins that block the activity of at least two proteins PDGF and VEGF receptors that are essential to the development of cancer. They interfere with the formation of new blood vessels in the area of the tumour, cutting off the supply of nutrients and oxygen which the tumour needs to grow and spread.

CITRUS FRUITS

Citrus fruits are not only a great source of Vitamin C, but they also contain two kinds of compounds called monoterpenes and flavanones which interfere with cancer cell growth and reduce inflammation which deprives cancer tumours stimulus for growth.

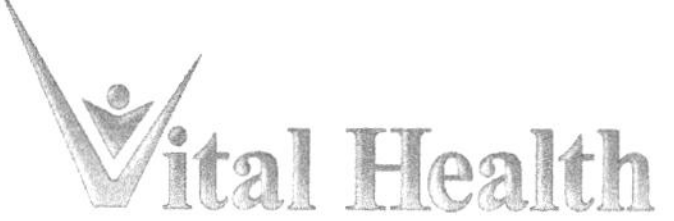

FATTY FISH

Fatty fish such as salmon, mackerel, herring and sardines have omega-3 that transforms into two polyunsaturated fats called docosahexaenoic acid (DHA) and eicosapentaenoic acid (EPA) which help defend against pathogens and cell tearing. Omega-3 has anti-inflammatory, anti-coagulant and anti-proliferative effects on cells of the body.

SEAWEED

Seaweed is rich in nutrients such as minerals like iodine, potassium, iron and calcium. Seaweed contains 10 times the calcium in cow's milk and five times the iron than spinach. The main types of seaweed are Nori, which comes as dried thin sheets used for sushi, Kombu, used in soup stock, Wakame, which is dark green, tender, used in Miso soups and eaten as a seaweed salad. Another is Arame, used in salads, soups or other dishes. Dulse is grown in Ireland, Scotland, Wales and Iceland and also harvested in Canada's eastern region along the coast of New Brunswick. It is eaten dried as a snack with beer in these regions. They contain two compounds fuxcoxanthin and fucoidan which inhibit cancer growth in the breast and prostate.

MUSHROOMS

The most commonly known one is the button mushroom or a similar variety the Portobello mushroom. These are used in most of the kitchens in North America, Europe, China, etc. They contain proteins called lectins that slow the growth of cancer cells. Shitake, originally grown in China then refined in its cultivation in Japan, is known for its medicinal property lentinan, a complex sugar with a powerful anti-cancer effect. It actually causes regression in tumour size when supplemented with chemotherapy on patients with colon and stomach cancer. Oyster mushrooms also have anti-cancer properties against isolated tumour cells.

GREEN TEA

Green tea leaves contain one of the highest proportions of anti-cancer molecules. One-third of the weight of the tea leaves are made up of catechins which are molecules that fight and prevent the development of cancer cells. Studies have shown that regular consumption of green tea greatly decreases the risk of certain types of cancer, predominantly those of the bladder and prostate. One of the most important catechins is EGCG which blocks mechanisms used by cancer cells to reproduce and invade surrounding tissue. It prevents the cancer cells from forming new networks of blood vessels by angiogenesis. Japanese green teas have higher levels of catechins. Three daily cups of the tea gives you optimum levels to protect against cancer.

RED WINE

Red wine contains thousands of phytochemical compounds. One of these, called resveratrol, can act simultaneously on multiple phases of cancer tumour development. It prevents both the forming of new cancer cells and the growth of mature cancer cells already present. Consume red wine in moderation because of the alcohol content. One glass a day with meals is adequate.

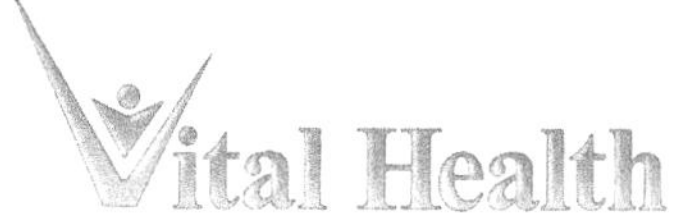

HERBS AND SPICES

Research has shown that herbs and spices contain molecules that reduce the production of cox-2, a principal enzyme used by cancer cells for inflammation. Turmeric and ginger seem to play an important role in preventing several types of cancer, especially colon cancer. Also, parsley and celery have high amounts of a compound called apigenin, a polyphenol which affects the cancer cells and angiogenesis indirectly by decreasing the inflammatory processes.

Here are the spices that have anti-cancer properties:

Turmeric
Ginger
Mint
Thyme
Marjoram
Oregano
Basil
Rosemary
Parsley
Coriander
Chervil
Fennel
Cumin

GOOD INTESTINAL BACTERIA

The main good bacteria lactobacilli and bifidobacteria causes increased activity of immune cells in our body and reduces inflammation which decreases the progression of cancer tumours. They also prevent the excessive growth of harmful bacteria.[92]

CRUCIFEROUS VEGETABLES

Cabbage is one of the vegetable belonging to this category along with such vegetables as broccoli, cauliflower, kale, Brussell sprouts and bok choy. These vegetables contain high amounts of glucosinolate which is a powerful anticancer molecules. It blocks many of the substances that can alter a cell's DNA, causing damage to the cell which gives rise to growth of tumours. Therefore, you should have at least three servings of these vegetables per week to keep the body at its optimal cancer prevention state.[93]

GARLIC FAMILY

Onions, garlic, leeks, shallots and chives are part of the Allium Sativum family. They carry a compound alliin which transforms into allicin a very unstable molecule that decomposes into about 30 compounds that have anti-cancer properties. These molecules are activated when these vegetables are crushed. They eliminate toxic substances from the body that attack our DNA which then causes multiple mutations leading to tumours. They act as border patrols in the first line of defence in the body. They also fight dormant microtumours and even force the cancer cells to destroy themselves.[94]

TOMATOES

Tomatoes contain lycopene, the compound which gives them their red colour. Lycopene also affects precancerous cell growth in the prostate. To allow lycopene to be more easily assimilated into the cells, you should cook the tomatoes in olive oil. This causes the lycopene to increase and absorb more readily into cells.[95]

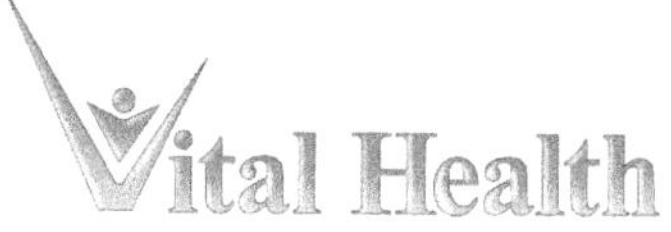

FLAX SEEDS

Flax seeds have a high amount of the complex compound Lignans. Two of these compounds, secoisolariciresinal and matairesinol, are converted by the intestinal bacteria into enterolactone and enterodiol molecules that interfere with the bonding of estrogens to breast cells. Flaxseeds also reduces chronic inflammation, thus decreasing precancerous cell growth. The seeds must be ground to increase absorption of omega-3 fatty acids and to help transform the lignans into active phytoestrogens.[96]

CANCER MEAL PLAN

UPON WAKING	CAL.	PROTEIN(G)	FAT(G)	CARBS.(G)
Drink 3 to 6 glasses of water upon the first hour and half of waking up (Note. 8 glasses of water if wrong combination of foods eaten the day before)				
4-8 oz fresh organic raspberries, blueberries with sprinkle of cinnamon or half a grapefruit	60	0.7	0	14
(Wait half hour to digest the fruit before breakfast)				
1 tbsp omega-3 oil or 3 capsules of fish oil, one powder capsule 50 mg vitamin B complex, 1 tsp Vitamin C powder, 1 capsule of probiotic supplement which has more than a billion good bacteria in it.				
2 level tbsp of liquid Daily Complete	130	0	13.5	0
BREAKFAST A (Note. you have the option of only having breakfast A or B in the mornings, hence your calorie total for the day will be less; however you can have both on days you are hungry)				
(Note. I suggest not to use milk with cereal but if you really find it hard to change, please at least get organic milk)				
8 oz. organic 2%, almond, rice milk or goat's milk	45	4.5		6
4 oz. seed cereal, organic steel cut oats, quinoa or millet with 2-3 tbsp of ground flax seeds added	65	1	1	11.5
8-12 oz. veg. / fruit. Juice (Note. 8 oz. organic spinach or cabbage, 4-6 carrots, apple and 4 inch chunk ginger)	69	1.9	0.35	16.1
BREAKFAST B 12 oz garden salad of sliced cucumbers, tomatoes, green pepper, fennel, parsley, oregano, mint, 8 oz. spinach or cabbage, two crushed garlic clove and ½ inch slice Spanish onion	50	3	0	7
1 tbsp olive oil & squeezed lemon juice	119		14	
2 eggs (poached, boiled or scrambled)	160	12	10	1
1 cup Japanese green tea				
Mid-morning snack (Note. optional if hungry)				
1 c of Pure Trim shake	86	14.6	1.3	4
(Note. Recipe for 3 cup protein shake: 2.5 cups of water, 1 banana, 4 oz. fresh or frozen strawberries, ½ pack Pure Trim)				

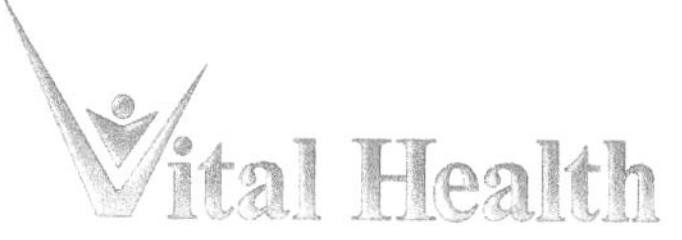

LUNCH (Note. drink 1.5 to 2 cups of water)				
4 oz. organic wild salmon baked, broiled or BBQ	208	30.6	8	0
8 oz. broccoli, Brussell sprouts, green beans, kale, or cauliflower, etc., with a ½ tsp of sea salt, ground pepper	40	4.5	0.5	7.5
12 oz cabbage and spinach salad with 1 tbsp olive oil & lemon juice and 3 oz of wakame salad	249	5	22	10.7
1 cup Japanese green tea				
MID-NOON SNACK (Note. drink 1.5 to 2 cups of water)				
4 oz raspberries, blue berries (Note. wait 30 minutes then eat protein snack)	20	0.3	Tr	4.6
½oz almonds	52	1.7	4.5	2
SUPPER (Note. drink 1.5 to 2 cups of water)				
8 oz organic squash or tomato soup	72	2	2	12
4 oz of mackerel, salmon, herring or sardines				
(Note: can top with tbsp of home-made sea food sauce of horse radish, tomato sauce and brown sugar)	226	24	14.6	0
8 oz. broccoli, Brussell sprouts, kale, or cauliflower, etc., with a ½ tsp of sea salt & pepper	40	4.5	0.5	7.5
12 oz. salad with 1 tbsp olive oil & lemon juice and 3 oz of wakame salad	249	5	22	10.7
EVENING SNACK 1 cup Japanese green tea				
4oz. fresh raspberries, blue berries and black berries				
(Note. wait 30 minutes then eat carb snack)	20	0.3	Trace	4.6
4 oz. low fat organic plain yogurt	72	6	2	8
TOTALS:	**2032**	**121.6**	**116.25**	**127.2**

Hypothyroidism

The thyroid is located in the front of the neck, made up of two halves that lie on each side of the trachea (windpipe), joined together by some thyroid tissue called isthmus. It looks after metabolism of the body, weight control, growth, digestion, body temperature, reflexes and heart beat. Hypothyroidism (underactive thyroid) is the most common problem which is caused by usually Hashimoto's disease, where the body's own immune system attacks healthy thyroid tissue. Males get it sometimes, but it is a huge problem with females. Studies show almost one in 10 females over the age of 65 have early stage hypothyroidism and this can usually be detected by a blood test. A significant number of cases, however, will have symptoms of thyroid imbalance even though blood tests show normal levels of thyroid hormones.[97]

Common symptoms are severe fatigue, enlarged thyroid (goiter), unexplained weight gain, chronic cold hands and feet, chronic constipation, dry skin, brittle nails, hair loss, depression and memory loss. Some of the causes of this disease are from radiation poisoning, excess estrogen from hormone replacement drugs like Premarin, oral contraceptives, hormone-mimicking chemicals in the environment, such as chemicals used in plastic bottles, Tupperware, etc.

One of the main toxins that contribute towards this disease in our environment is fluoride which is in our water, bottled drinks, foods, and toothpaste. Fluoride reduces iodine in your system. Hypothyroidism was not a major known problem in North America until municipalities began to fluoridate their water systems in the late 1940s. The pituitary gland located in our brain controls the functioning of all glands and it soaks up fluoride in the body readily like a sponge. When this happens, the gland stops producing the TSH hormone that stimulates the thyroid, allowing hypothyroidism to occur. Unfortunately, even if you take in iodine into the body it will not remedy this condition if the pituitary is full of fluoride. Fluoride is also in the air. We breathe it from the discharge of coal-burning plants still in operation. European water systems are 98 percent fluoride free. Hong Kong has had fluoridated water since 1961 and hypothyroidism is high there. When you cook with fluoridated water in aluminum or Teflon coated pans and pots you are releasing both aluminum and fluoride into your body. The aluminum content of your food increases by 800 times. The high rate of Alzheimer's disease in North America can be traced to fluoridated water, aluminum and Teflon cooking pans.

I have provided a chart created by Linda Tanguay (Certified Bio-Feedback Consultant) indicating all the symptoms of hypothyroidism and foods that inhibit thyroid hormone production, hence blocking iodine absorption leading to hypothyroidism. These are called goitrogenic foods. The chart indicates various levels of the goitrogenic affect of some foods.

Also, for the hypothyroid meal plan that is given, you may have to adjust the portion size of vegetables, fish, fruit, etc. based on activity levels and how hungry you are. For example, instead of eating 4 oz of fish, have 6-8 ounces. The total calorie count of the meal plan will vary somewhat from person to person. For a small female, the calorie total may only be around 1700 calories. If you are not hungry at mid-morning, it is not necessary to have the Pure Trim shake. Breakfast A and Breakfast B are options of what you can have for breakfast. If you are an athlete, serious runner or bodybuilder you will need a higher calorie meal in the morning and may need to have both breakfasts A and B in the morning.

HYPERTHYROIDISM

In this case, a person's thyroid produces too much thyroid hormone causing the metabolism of the body to increase, causing swelling of the thyroid gland, weight-loss, sweating and rapid heartbeat. Usually medication is needed to control this condition. However, it does help to avoid foods that are rich in iodine such as seaweed, kelp and sea salt. Also because of the accelerated rate of metabolism, caffeine and refined sugar foods should be avoided as it further aggravates the condition. People with hypothyroidism have to avoid eating thyroid suppressing foods, like cauliflower, kale, broccoli, peaches, soybeans and turnips which can help their condition. Furthermore, you should eat foods that are high in calcium and rich in antioxidants. Because of their high metabolism, people with this condition can deplete their nutrients fast, especially vitamins B12 and D. So they may need to take extra B12 and D supplements. [98]

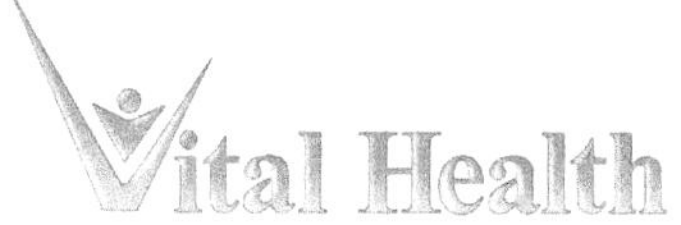

HYPOTHYROIDISM CHART

SYMPTOMS: Fatigue, sluggishness, increased sensitivity to cold, constipation, pale/dry skin, puffy face, hoarse voice, elevated blood cholesterol level, unexplained weight gain, muscle aches/tenderness and stiffness, pain/stiffness or swelling in joints, muscle weakness, heavier than normal menstrual periods, brittle fingernails and hair, depression.

GOITROGENS: foods that inhibit the production of thyroid hormones because they interfere with iodine absorption. Cooking these foods reduces their potentially adverse affects (except soy), therefore, eating limited amounts cooked, twice a week max, is advised for their other health benefits.

AVOID	Cruciferous Veg. (Brassica)	Fluoride	Chloride or Bromide	Caffeine (suppressant)	Goitrogen Level	SEEK	Iodine mcg/100g Food women need 120 mcg Iodine / day	Stimulant
Bamboo Shoots						Avocado		X
Bok Choy	X					Bananas		X
Broccoli	X				***	Beans		
Brussell sprouts	X					Coconut/Coconut Oil		X
Cabbage	X				***	Cod	110	
Canola /								
Grapeseed	X					Cod Liver Oil	838	
Cauliflower	X				***	Egg (1 boiled)	24	
Chocolate				X		Flax Seeds		
Coffee				X		Garlic		X
Cola				X		Haddock	250	
Collard Greens	X					Herring	29	
Gluten						Lobster	100	
Green Tea		X	X			Mayonnaise	36	
Horse radish						Mackerel	140	

Kale	X					Meat	26	
Kohlrabi	X					Mussels	140	
Millet					***	Nuts		
Mustard	X				**	Oats/Oatmeal		
Peaches					*	Onion		
Peanuts						Oysters	60	
Pears					*	Parsley		
Pine nuts					*	Potato (1 med baked w / peel)	60	
Radish						Prawns	21	
Rapini	X					Pumpkin Seeds		
Rutabaga	X					Raisins		
Soy					****	Salmon (Atlantic)	76	
Spinach					*	Salt (1/4 tsp iodized)	105	
Strawberry					*	Seaweed (1/4 cup Kelp)	415	
Sweet Potatoes						Shrimp	100	
Tea				X		Sushi	100	
Textured Vegetable Protein						Tuna	30	
Turnip	X				**	Watermelon		X
White flour						Yogurt (1 cup low fat)	87[99]	

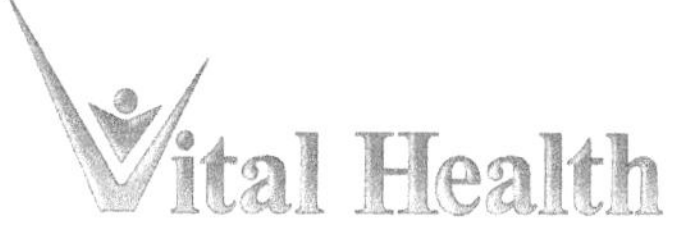

HYPOTHYROIDISM MEAL PLAN

UPON WAKING	CAL.	PROTEIN(G)	FAT(G)	CARBS.(G)
Drink 3 to 6 glasses of water upon the first hour and half of waking up (Note. 8 glasses of water if wrong combination of foods eaten the day before)				
4-84 - 8 oz fresh watermelon with half banana, sprinkle with cinnamon and ½ doz. raisins	60	0.7	0	14
(Note. wait half hour to digest the fruit before breakfast)				
1 tbsp omega-3 oil or 3 capsules of fish oil, 1-2 capsule of cod liver oil, powder capsule 50 mg vitamin B complex, 1 tsp Vitamin C powder, and 1 capsule of probiotic supplement which has more than a billion good bacteria in it.				
2 level tbsp of liquid Daily Complete	130	0	13.5	0
BREAKFAST A (Note. you have the option of only having breakfast A or B in the mornings, hence your calorie total for the day will be less; however you can have both on days you are hungry)				
(Note. I suggest not to use milk with cereal but if you really find it hard to change, please at least get organic milk)				
8 oz. organic 2% milk, coconut or almond milk	45	4.5		6
4 oz. seed cereal or steel cut oatmeal with 2-3 tbsp of flax seeds added	65	1	1	11.5
8-12 oz. veg. / fruit. Juice (4-6 carrots, apple, quarter beet, celery and 1 inch chunk ginger), 1 cup herbal tea	69	1.9	0.35	16.1
BREAKFAST B 8 oz salad of sliced cucumbers, tomatoes, green pepper, parsley, oregano, romaine lettuce, ½ inch slice Spanish onion, crushed garlic & ¼ sea salt	50	3	0	7
2 eggs (poached, boiled or scrambled)	160	12	10	1
LUNCH (Note. drink 1.5 to 2 cups of water)				
4 oz. haddock, mackerel, lobster, cod, or salmon baked, broiled or BBQ	208	30.6	8	0
8 oz. green beans, white potato, carrots, and zucchini with a ¼ tsp of sea salt, ground pepper	40	4.5	0.5	7.5

8 oz salad of romaine lettuce, tomato, celery, bell pepper and cucumber with 1 tbsp olive oil & lemon juice, ¼ sea salt, with 3 oz wakame seaweed salad	214	6	20	16
MID-NOON SNACK (Note. drink 1.5 to 2 cups of water)				
4-8 oz raspberries, blueberries (Note. wait 30 minutes to digest fruit then eat protein snack)	60	.7		14
4 oz. plain organic low fat yogurt, ½ tsp maple syrup, ½ oz almonds	222.5	15.5	13	26.5
SUPPER (Note. drink 1.5 to 2 cups of water)				
8 oz. organic soup tomato soup	72	2	2	12
4 oz of mackerel, haddock, lobster, salmon or shrimp				
(Note: tbsp of organic BBQ sauce can be used)	226	24	14.6	0
12 oz steamed zucchini, green beans, Swiss chard	40	4.5	0.5	7.5
3 oz of wakame seaweed salad	45	3	.6	9
12 oz salad with 1 tbsp vinaigrette	50	3	0	7
EVENING SNACK 1 cup herbal tea				
13 five Mary's Organic crackers (gluten free)	140	3	5	21
TOTALS:	**1896.5**	**119.9**	**89.05**	**176.1**

Candida Albicans Infection

Candida Albicans is a common yeast fungus that occurs naturally in the vagina, the mouth, digestive tract and on the scalp. When it increases to abnormal levels, it becomes a problem and health issue. When overactive in the vagina, women experience soreness, itchiness and white thick discharge, and can experience sugar cravings, fatigue, insomnia, puffy eyes, urinary tract infections, depression and rectal itching. Some of the main causes of an overgrowth of Candida are from use of antibiotics which kill bad and good bacteria. Good bacteria is needed to control the Candida, but it cannot because it has been depleted. Poor diet consisting of excess sugar, dairy, tea, and coffee increases urine sugar which encourages the yeast growth. During pregnancy, estrogen levels increase which increase the sugar content (and pH level) of the vagina. This becomes an ideal environment for the yeast to grow. Women with diabetes also tend to have higher sugar levels in their urine because of raised sugar levels in their blood, and are therefore susceptible to the yeast growth. Stress causes the immune system to drop, making women vulnerable to yeast infections.

NATURAL REMEDIES

One of the ways to kill Candida is to spoon apple cider vinegar and yogurt into the vagina. Adding a tablespoon of flaxseed oil to daily meals will help prevent yeast infection.

MORE REMEDIES:

- **Olive Leaf Extract** – natural anti-fungal properties protects against parasites and viral infections
- **Kolorex** – herbal extract which contains Horopito herb that kills Candida
- **Caprylic Acid** – acts as an anti-fungal, cleansing the digestive system, best taken as a enteric-coated time-release capsule
- **Tanalbit** – kills off bacteria and fungus without harming the good bacteria; acts as a natural antiseptic and prevents Candida colonization
- **Citrus Seeds & Grapefruit extract** – acts as natural anti-fungal against Candida; grapefruit extract can interfere with medication so consult your doctor
- **Pau D'Arco** – is a natural antifungal formula that helps to clear the body of toxins and enhances the immune system
- **Oregano Oil** – Studies show it is effective against 30 different bacteria growths and Candida
- **Douching** – washing the vagina with fluid mixture, using lactobacillus or yogurt
- **Stress Management** – manage stress levels by decreasing workload; get enough sleep, fit in 30 minutes a day for a brisk walk and exercise

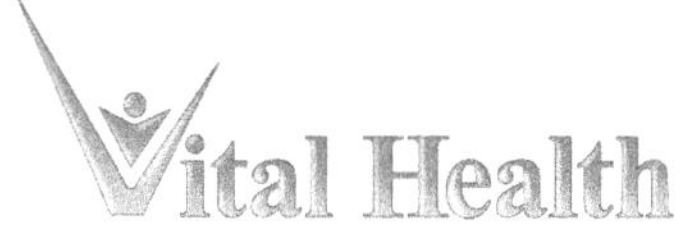

CANDIDA DIET PLAN

One of the main ways to eliminate Candida is through the foods you consume. If your symptoms are severe, then you want to eliminate certain foods for three weeks and slowly re-introduce some of the foods when the symptoms are clear. Refined carbohydrates, processed foods and high sugar foods should be eliminated from the diet permanently and only consumed as a treat once in awhile. Some dairy, like cheese, organic goat's milk and Tzatziki, can be consumed moderately, a couple times a week. This will keep the internal environment of the digestive tract from further re-growth of the Candida. Again, you may have to adjust your portion sizes of the meals and snacks according to how hungry you are and the amount of fuel you need for your activity level.

Here is the list of the vegetables you can have:

Asparagus
Artichoke
Organic Lettuce
Bean sprouts
Broccoli
Parsley
Beets
Brussels sprouts
Spinach
Cauliflower
Eggplant
Turnips
Organic Spinach
Turnip
Watercress
Organic Kale
Onions
Cucumber
Rhubarb
Sauerkraut
Bok Choy
Summer squash
Tomatoes and tomato juice
Zucchini
Alfalfa sprouts
Bell peppers
Cabbage
Organic Celery
Chicory

GRAINS

Since most grain foods are in the form of breads and baked goods that have yeast in it, it's best to avoid them during an anti-Candida diet. Stick to eating grains in their natural state such as a cereal or as a complex carbohydrate part of a meal. Keep to a serving size of half a cup per day of any of the following:

Brown rice
Wild rice
Pot Barley
Organic Steel Cut Oats
Quinoa
Millet

BEANS

Beans are a great source of protein and are rich in nutrients and helpful in controlling blood sugar levels. Have about two to three daily half-cup servings during this diet from any of the following on the list:

Kidney beans
Lentils
Lima beans
Pinto beans
Soybeans
Split peas
Black-eyed peas
Garbanzo beans

NUTS & SEEDS

Nuts and seeds are an excellent source of essential fatty acids, protein, Vitamin E and minerals. Even though they are high in calories, they are low on the glycemic index and they keep you full longer. Have up to three servings of seeds and three servings of nuts a day in the anti-Candida diet. The following is a list of options with their serving size:

Almonds: 8
Brazil nuts: 2 large or 3 small
Flax seeds: 2 tbsp
Hazelnuts: 4 large or 6 small
Macadamia nuts: 4 large
Pecans: 2 large

Olives: 5 small
Pine nuts: 2 tbsp
Pumpkin seeds: 2 tbsp
Sesame seeds: 2 tbsp
Sunflower seeds: 2 tbsp
Walnuts: 5 small

PROTEIN

Have a small servings of meat, fish and eggs during this diet phase. Choose any 2-3 of these options from the list as your protein for the day:

Organic Free Range Beef: 4oz
Free Range Eggs: 1-2
Wild Fish: 4oz
Lamb: 4oz
Organic Chicken/Turkey: 4oz

FRUITS

In severe cases of Candida, you need to eliminate all fruits for the three weeks of the diet. Then once the Candida clears, you can slowly introduce some fruits back into the diet. For those with normal levels of Candida and are not suffering with too many symptoms, one to two portions of fruit a day can be tolerated in the amounts indicated.[100]

Apple: 1
Blackberries: 1 cup
Cranberries: 1 cup
Apricots: 4
Strawberries: 1 cup
Raspberries: 1 cup
Banana: 1
Cherries: 20
Dates: 3
Grapefruit: 1
Grapes: 15
Orange: 1
Papayas: 1 cup
Peaches: 1
Pineapple: 1 cup
Prunes: 4
Tangerines: 2

Fruits to Avoid:

Melons	Cantaloupe	Dried figs
Watermelons	Raisins	Dried apricots

CANDIDA MEAL PLAN

UPON WAKING	CAL.	PROTEIN(G)	FAT(G)	CARBS.(G)
Drink 3 to 6 glasses of water upon the first hour and half of waking up (Note. 8 glasses of water if wrong combination of foods eaten the day before)				
4-8 oz organic apple, strawberries or grapefruit	60	0.7	0	14
(Note. wait half hour to digest the fruit before breakfast) 1 tbsp omega-3 oil or 3 capsules of fish oil, one powder capsule 50 mg vitamin B complex, 1 tsp Vitamin C powder, 1 capsule of probiotic supplement which has more than a billion good bacteria in it. 2 level tbsp of liquid Daily Complete	130	0	13.5	0
BREAKFAST A (Note. you cannot use milk with cereal)				
8 oz. organic unsweetened almond milk or rice milk	45	4.5		6
4 oz. seed cereal, steel cut oatmeal or millet	65	1	1	11.5
8-12 oz. veg. juice (4-6 cucumber, bell pepper, celery, 2-3 kale leaves, spinach, beets and 1 inch chunk ginger), 1 cup herbal tea	69	1.9	0.35	16.1
BREAKFAST B (Note. you have the option of only having breakfast A or B in the mornings, hence your calorie total for the day will be less; however you can have both on days you are hungry)				
12 oz garden salad of sliced cucumbers, tomatoes, green pepper, parsley, oregano, 8 oz. romaine lettuce, and ½ inch slice Spanish onion,	130	4	8	10.7
1 tbsp olive oil & squeezed lemon juice	119	1	14	
2 free range eggs (poached, boiled or scrambled)	160	12	10	1

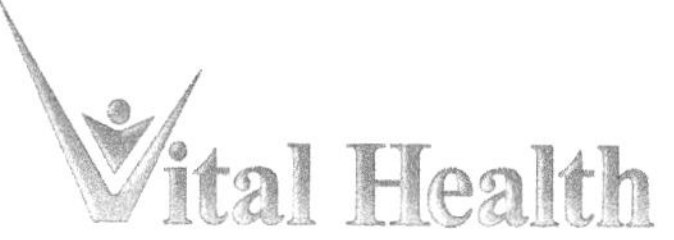

LUNCH (Note. drink 1.5 to 2 cups of water)				
4 oz free range beef, chicken, lamb or wild salmon baked, broiled or BBQ	208	30.6	8	0
8 oz broccoli, cauliflower, Brussell sprouts or zucchini with a ¼ tsp of sea salt, ground pepper	40	4.5	0.5	7.5
12 oz salad romaine lettuce, tomato, celery, bell pepper and cucumber salad with 1 tbsp vinaigrette	50	3	0	7
MID-NOON SNACK (Note. drink 1.5 to 2 cups of water)				
4-8 oz raspberries, blue berries (Note. wait 30 minutes then eat protein or carb snack)	60	0.7		14
4 oz organic oat meal with 8 oz almond milk	116	3.5	6.5	15.5
SUPPER (Note. drink 1.5 to 2 cups of water)				
8 oz organic squash or tomato soup	72	2	2	12
8 oz wild fish, organic chicken, free range beef, lamb or meat stew (Note: use fresh spices like garlic, thyme, parsley)	373	45	12	1
16 oz broccoli, cauliflower, Brussell sprouts, turnip or zucchini with a ¼ tsp of sea salt, ground pepper	160	18	2	30
12 oz. salad with 1 tbsp vinaigrette	50	3	0	7
EVENING SNACK 1 cup herbal tea				
4oz. fresh raspberries, blue berries or black berries (Note. wait 30 minutes then eat protein snack)	20	0.3	Trace	4.6
12 unsalted roasted almonds	78	2.5	6.7	3
TOTALS:	**2005**	**138.2**	**84.55**	**160.9**

Crohns

This is an inflammatory bowel disease where inflammation of the intestinal tract occurs. It can take place in your mouth, esophagus, stomach, small intestine, large intestine (colon), rectum, and anus. In many cases, people mistake the symptoms of Crohn's disease for lactose intolerance, irritable bowel syndrome or intestinal parasite. Since this is a chronic disease, the symptoms may go away for long periods of time then come back suddenly.

Here are some of the main symptoms to watch for:

- Severe abdominal pain, usually right after eating and around the navel, lower right abdomen or both
- Frequent diarrhea (with or without blood)
- Rectal bleeding (blood and /or mucus in the stool)
- Rectal urgency (frequent, urgent bowel movements)
- Weight loss (usually due to the discomfort after eating or also due to nutritional deficiency)
- Increased gas
- A persistent lack of energy
- Firm, grapefruit sized swelling in the lower right abdomen that's usually painful to touch (found in about 25% of Crohn's patients)

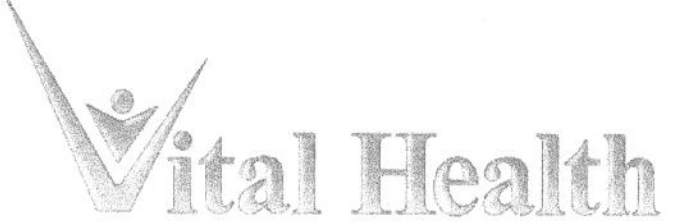

- Perianal disease (a fistula which may include one or more abscesses and skin tags around the anus that affects 25% of Crohn's patients)
- Children who do not grow at proper rates

It is easy to sometimes misinterpret the symptoms. These symptoms may indicate the person is suffering from another condition:

- Abdominal pain, vomiting or diarrhea that clears up between 36 to 48 hours after a diet of clear liquids, bland food such as soda crackers, rice or toasted bread.
- Abdominal pain, diarrhea, and fever relieved by over-the-counter medications such as Pepto-Bismol, Imodium A-D, or Tylenol
- Symptoms that occur after eating dairy foods like milk, ice-cream, cheese, or yogurt and they go away after these foods are removed from the diet
- Symptoms may be linked to stress or may be irritable bowel syndrome (IBS)
- Alternating diarrhea and constipation

You should go and see a doctor if you think you have it to get a proper diagnosis. However, don't be surprised if all you get is prescription drugs from your doctor which is a Band-Aid solution. I believe the source of much of this disease comes from the diet we, in the West, consume. Our western diet, unfortunately, is made up of eating too many foods that cause our body to use hydrochloric acid to digest our food instead of enzymes and bile. Bile and enzymes don't cause damage to the delicate tissues of the esophagus, throat, intestinal cilia and mucosal lining. I believe it's mainly the wrong food and drink, medications, and toxins causing the high acidity which eventually eat away at the intestinal lining that lead to digestive diseases such as Crohn's.[101]

Even though there is no known cure, Crohn's can be managed quite well and much of the symptoms eliminated through correcting eating habits. The main way this is done is by eating enough raw foods high in enzymes and foods that cause bile to be secreted to digest food instead of hydrochloric acid. The following is a sample meal plan that can be used if you are suffering from Crohn's.

CROHN'S MEAL PLAN

UPON WAKING	CAL.	PROTEIN(G)	FAT(G)	CARBS.(G)
Drink 3 to 6 glasses of water upon the first hour and half of waking up (Note. 8 glasses of water if wrong combination of foods eaten the day before)				
4-8 oz organic apple or half banana	60	0.7	0	14
(Note. wait half hour to digest the fruit before breakfast)				
1 tbsp omega-3 oil or 3 capsules of fish oil, one powdered capsule of 50 mg vitamin B complex, 1 tsp Vitamin C powder, and 1 capsule of probiotic supplement which has more than a billion good bacteria in it.				
2 level tbsp of liquid Daily Complete	130	0	13.5	0
BREAKFAST A (Note. you have the option of only having breakfast A or B in the mornings, hence your calorie total for the day will be less; however you can have both on days you are hungry)				
8 oz. organic unsweetened almond or rice milk	45	4.5		6
4-8 oz. steel cut organic well cooked oatmeal (you can even eat it during Crohn's symptom flare ups)	65	1	1	11.5
8-12 oz. veg. juice (4-6 carrots, quarter beet, celery, 2-3 Kale leaves and 1 inch chunk ginger), 1 cup herbal tea	69	1.9	0.35	16.1
BREAKFAST B 12 oz garden salad of sliced cucumbers, tomatoes, green pepper, parsley, oregano, romaine lettuce, and ½ inch slice Spanish onion & 1 tbsp vinaigrette	50	3	0	7
2 free range eggs (poached, boiled or scrambled)	160	12	10	1
LUNCH (Note. drink 1.5 to 2 cups of water)				
4 oz. haddock, mackerel, herring or salmon baked, broiled or BBQ (Note. Omega-3 in the fish helps with inflammation when the symptoms flare up from Crohns)	208	30.6	8	0
12 oz broccoli, cauliflower, Brussell sprouts, turnip or zucchini with a ¼ tsp of sea salt, ground pepper	30	2	0	7

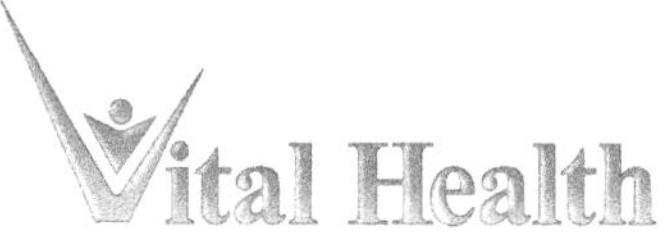

Bowl of romaine lettuce, tomato, celery, bell pepper and cucumber salad with 1 tbsp olive oil & lemon juice and add 3 oz wakame seaweed salad (Note. you can put in 1 oz of diced Swiss or mozzarella cheese)	214	6	20	16
MID-NOON SNACK (Note. drink 1.5 to 2 cups of water)				
4-8 oz raspberries, blue berries (Note. have applesauce or banana if there is a flare up instead)	60	.7		14
(Note. wait 30 minutes after having fruit then eat carb snack)				
4-8 oz cooked peeled potato, carrots, brown rice or rice pasta (Note. skin of the potato may aggravate inflammation if your Crohn's condition is severe)	176	4		41
SUPPER (Note. drink 1.5 to 2 cups of water)				
8 oz. organic squash or tomato soup	72	2	2	12
4 oz of wild mackerel, salmon, organic chicken, free range beef, or lamb (Note: use fresh garlic, thyme, and parsley)	226	24	14.6	0
12 oz carrots, zucchini, green beans, Swiss chard (Note. well cooked and soft)	40	4.5	0.5	7.5
12 oz. salad with tbsp of olive oil and lemon juice	249	5	22	10.7
EVENING SNACK (Note. choose one of the snack options and have the other on another day)				
1 cup herbal tea				
4 oz organic steel cut oat meal with 8 oz almond milk (Note. cook the oatmeal well so it is soft)	116	3.5	6.5	15.5
4 oz. fresh raspberries, blue berries or black berries and 4 oz of plain organic yogurt (Note. good bacteria in the yogurt can help in the recovery of the intestine)	92	12	4	20.6
TOTALS:	**2062**	**117.4**	**102.45**	**199.9**

102

Diverticulitis

This is a disease where small sacs develop along the wall of the colon from too much pressure on the weakened spots of the intestinal walls by gas, waste or liquid. This pressure is caused mainly from the straining that happens when people are constipated or their stool is too hard. Passing it out during elimination takes a lot of pressure and force. This condition is very common among people and occurs in 10 percent of the people over 40 and in 50 percent of the people over the age of 60. In about 20 percent of the people who have diverticulitis, rectal bleeding occurs and others experience infections in the sacs that develop. The infections occur when waste gets trapped inside the sacs causing bacteria to accumulate. The rectal bleeding occurs from chronic injury that happens to small blood vessels next to the diverticula (sacs that develop).

Most people don't show symptoms, however, when they show up, they can happen suddenly without warning. The symptoms usually come in the form of infection and inflammation. The symptoms can be alternating diarrhea and constipation, painful cramps, tenderness in the lower abdomen area, chills, and fever. People who do not have symptoms or complications need to have a high-fibre diet to prevent forming more diverticula. Complications can occur from this condition since it usually was caused from some sort of a perforation or tear in the intestinal wall. The waste can leak out of the intestines into surrounding abdominal areas causing problems such as peritonitis (painful infection of the abdominal cavity),

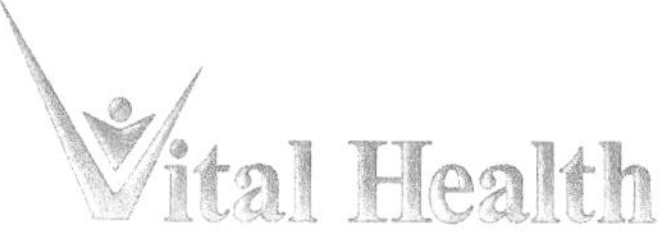

abscesses ("walled off" infections in the abdomen), and obstruction (blockages of the intestines).[103]

The lack of fibre is the main cause of diverticulitis because it causes slow transit time where it takes two to three times longer to pass through the colon. This then causes too much water absorption which results in a very dry stool that is difficult to pass, where forceful peristaltic contraction has to happen to move the stool along. During the process, pockets of the diverticula are produced from the pressure. However, a high-fibre diet of unrefined grains, raw fruits, and vegetables help prevent this from happening. The stools are two to three times as bulky and because of the higher fibre content they have absorbed more water, hence they are a softer stool that passes easily without much force during a bowel movement. During an acute stage of this condition, a liquid fast of fresh juices done in a juicing machine and teas are advised. Store bought juices are pasteurized so they do not have the nutrient and enzyme content, therefore should be avoided.

Here are the following juices that you can make with the juice machine for this condition:

- Carrot juice
- Carrot and lettuce juice
- Celery and lettuce
- Beet juice
- Watercress juice
- Grape juice
- Apple juice
- Slippery elm tea
- Comfrey tea
- Marshmallow tea
- Chlorophyll liquid or wheatgrass liquid drinks
- Spirulina liquid drinks

This liquid diet should be phased out as the painful symptoms disappear. Semi-solid food should slowly be introduced back into the diet. Papaya, mashed banana, steamed carrots, and baked yams are good choices. Still watch for any reactions. Once these foods are tolerated you can add other cooked, grated raw foods and pureed foods that are high in fibre. Also drink a minimum of about 8-10 glasses of water per day. Still avoid fruit skins, fruit and vegetables with small hard seeds such as tomatoes, cucumbers, figs, strawberries, raspberries, guavas, etc. Then start to add grains and proteins like well cooked brown rice and quinoa which should be chewed many times. Once these foods are tolerated, you can proceed to include all natural unrefined foods. Getting the body used to a high fibre diet takes about six to eight weeks. In most cases, as long as you remain on this kind of eating you can remain symptom-free. Changing the diet is 90 percent of the solution. [104]

DIVERTICULITIS MEAL PLAN

UPON WAKING	CAL.	PROTEIN(G)	FAT(G)	CARBS.(G)
Drink 3 to 6 glasses of water upon the first hour and half of waking up (Note. 8 glasses of water if wrong combination of foods eaten the day before)				
One ripe peach peeled, cut up (Note. also can have nectarines, oranges, plums, papaya or grapefruit)	87	1	0	10
(Note. wait half hour to digest the fruit before breakfast)				
1 tbsp omega-3 oil or 3 capsules of fish oil, one powdered capsule of 50 mg vitamin B complex, 1 tsp Vitamin C powder, and 1 capsule of probiotic supplement which has more than a billion good bacteria in it.	130	0	13.5	0
2 level tbsp of liquid Daily Complete				
BREAKFAST A 8 oz organic goat's milk, almond or rice milk	121	8	5	12
4 oz organic corn flakes, well cooked oat meal, cream of wheat, couscous or millet (Note. have fibre foods that help to keep stool soft, as it absorbs water so eliminating becomes much easier)	65	1	1	11.5
8-12 oz. veg. juice with no pulp (4-6 carrots, quarter beet and spinach) and 1 cup herbal tea	69	1.9	0.35	16.1

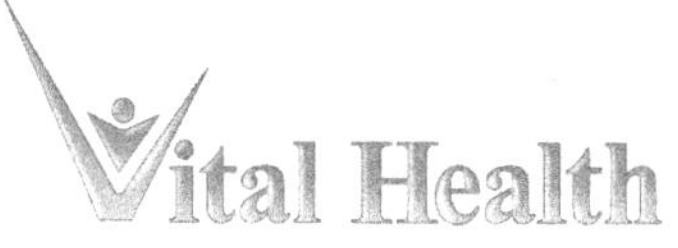

BREAKFAST B (Note. you have the option of only having breakfast A or B in the mornings, hence your calorie total for the day will be less; however you can have both on days you are hungry)				
12 oz salad of peeled and seedless sliced cucumbers, zucchini, lettuce and tomatoes and ¼ avocado [105] & 1 tbsp olive oil & lemon juice	249	5	22	10.7
2 free range eggs (poached, boiled or scrambled)	160	12	10	1
LUNCH (Note. drink 1.5 to 2 cups of water)				
4 oz. mackerel, salmon, beef baked, broiled or BBQ	208	30.6	8	0
8 oz. green beans, carrots, cauliflower, asparagus, eggplant, parsnips, rutabagas, squash or zucchini well cooked with a ¼ tsp of sea salt, ground pepper	40	4.5	0.5	7.5
12 oz of salad of peeled, seedless sliced cucumbers, zucchini, lettuce and tomatoes & 1 tbsp vinaigrette	50	3	0	7
MID-NOON SNACK Drink 1.5 to 2 cups of water before meal				
Half of one peeled, cooked sweet potato	172	3		40
SUPPER (Note. drink 1.5 to 2 cups of water)				
8 oz. organic squash or tomato soup	72	2	2	12
4 oz of broiled organic chicken, free range lamb, beef or wild fish				
(Note: use fresh spices like garlic, thyme, parsley)	226	24	14.6	0
12 oz. green beans and carrots, well cooked with a ¼ tsp of sea salt, ground pepper (Note. also can have these choices: cauliflower, asparagus, eggplant, parsnips, rutabagas, squash or zucchini) [106]	40	4.5	0.5	7.5
12 oz of salad of peeled, seedless sliced cucumbers, zucchini, lettuce and tomatoes & tbsp vinaigrette [107]	50	3	0	7
EVENING SNACK 4 oz plain organic yogurt with half a fresh peeled and cored pear and one cup of herbal tea	121	7	3	20.5
TOTALS:	**1860**	**110.5**	**80.45**	**162.8**

Irritable Bowel Syndrome

Irritable Bowel Syndrome (IBS) is the abbreviated term to describe this bowel issue that is a problem among a significant portion of the population in the West. Usually people experience abdominal pain, discomfort from change in bowel movements, excessive gas, bloating, diarrhea or constipation.

The best way to treat IBS is through proper diet and avoiding certain foods on a regular basis. Furthermore, physical therapy can be used along with stress management. As studies have shown, there is a brain-to-bowel connection as mentioned earlier. The enteric nervous system (ENS) runs along the gastrointestinal tract and every class of neurotransmitter found in the brain is also found in the ENS. The central nervous system (CNS), which is made up of the brain and the spinal column, is connected with the ENS through the vagus nerve which is the longest of the cranial nerves. The ENS also has the same number of neurotransmitters as the brain, about a hundred million. Therefore there are two types of nerves that control the digestive system. They are the extrinsic and intrinsic nerves. The extrinsic nerves are from the brain and the spinal cord and they release the neurotransmitters acetycholine and adrenaline that cause the muscles of the digestive organs to perform their peristalsis wave of relaxing and contracting. The intrinsic nerves are embedded within the walls of the digestive tract and organs. They regulate the release of various substances that regulate the speed at which the food moves through the system and the production of digestive juices needed for different foods passing through.[108] Therefore, when you control

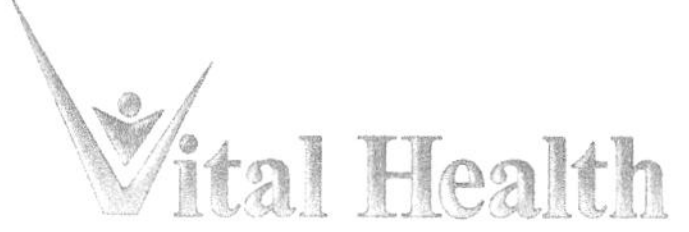

your stress level, emotions and are more calm, you have peace and harmony in your life style, the bowel functions and digestion also respond. This is due to the fact that the ENS is also connected to your brain. Therefore, less IBS symptoms may occur.[109]

Each person with IBS is sensitive to different foods and has different triggers that aggravate their system. However, these are the main foods that you need to stay away from on a regular basis.

You need to avoid the following

high fat foods

alcohol	spicy foods
caffeinated coffee and tea	beans
cabbage	broccoli
Brussels sprouts	bagels
peas	cauliflower
fried foods	onions

These can cause discomfort in most people with IBS where they will experience bloating, gas, and abdominal pain. It's important to avoid or eat less of the foods that trigger the IBS symptoms. Avoid or eat fewer foods that the small intestine has trouble absorbing. These foods increase fluid in the bowels and create more gas. This leads to slower digestion speed due to bloating and the result is gas, pain and diarrhea.

Try to eat less of these foods:

Milk	Apricots
Yogurt	Blackberries
Cottage cheese and ricotta cheese	Cherries
Pudding	Nectarines
Ice-cream	Pears
Apples	Peaches

Mangoes
Watermelon
Artichokes
Broccoli
Beetroot
Cauliflower
Garlic
Mushrooms
Onions
Snow peas
Wheat and rye
Legumes
Corn syrup products
Sweeteners such as honey, agave nectar, sorbitol, etc.

Eat more of these foods that have less trigger effects:

Lactose-free rice, almond and coconut milk
Lactose-free yogurt
Hard cheeses
Bananas
Blueberries
Cantaloupe
Grapefruit
Honeydew melon
Kiwi
Lemon
Oranges
Strawberries
Bamboo shoots
Bean sprouts
Bok choy
Carrots
Cucumbers
Eggplant
Ginger
Lettuce
Olives
Parsnips
Potatoes
Turnips
Beef
Chicken
Fish
Eggs
Tofu
Almonds, macadamia and pine nuts
Walnuts
Oats and oat bran
Rice bran
Gluten-free pasta
Corn flour
Quinoa

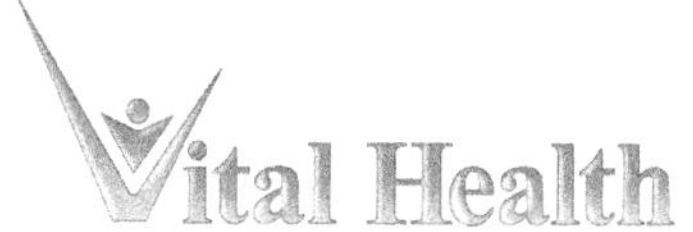

The following sample meal plan for IBS will have many of these foods listed in the meals.[110]

IRRITABLE BOWEL SYNDROME MEAL PLAN

UPON WAKING	CAL.	PROTEIN(G)	FAT(G)	CARBS.(G)
Drink 3 to 6 glasses of water upon the first hour and half of waking up (Note. 8 glasses of water if wrong combination of foods eaten the day before)				
4-8 oz fresh fruit with sprinkle of cinnamon (Note. banana, apples, nectarines, berries, etc.)	50	0.5	Trace	26
(Note. wait half hour to digest the fruit before breakfast) 1 tbsp omega-3 oil or 3 capsules of fish oil, one powdered capsule of 50 mg vitamin B complex, 1 tsp Vitamin C powder, and 1 capsule of probiotic supplement which has more than a billion good bacteria in it. 2 level tbsp of liquid Daily Complete	130	0	13.5	0
BREAKFAST A (Note. I suggest not to use milk but if you really find it hard to change, please at least get organic milk)				
8 oz. organic almond or rice milk	45	4.5		6
4 oz organic oatmeal, quinoa, millet, or seed cereal	65	1	1	11.5
8-12 oz. veg. juice (Note. 4-6 carrots, quarter beet, celery, 2-3 Kale leaves and 1 inch chunk ginger, made fresh in Juice Machine), 1 cup herbal tea	69	1.9	0.35	16.1
BREAKFAST B (Note. you have the option of only having breakfast A or B in the mornings, hence your calorie total for the day will be less; however you can have both on days you are hungry)				
12 oz garden salad of sliced cucumbers, tomatoes, green pepper, parsley, oregano, romaine and carrots	50	3	0	7
1 tbsp olive oil & squeezed lemon juice	119	1	14	

2 free range eggs (poached, boiled or scrambled)	160	12	10	1
LUNCH				
(Note. drink 1.5 to 2 cups of water)				
4 oz. haddock, mackerel, organic chicken, free range beef or salmon baked, broiled or BBQ	208	30.6	8	0
8 oz. steamed green beans, bok choy, parsnips, and zucchini with a ¼ tsp of sea salt, ground pepper	40	4.5	0.5	7.5
12 oz salad of romaine lettuce, tomato, celery, bell pepper and cucumber with 1 tbsp vinaigrette	50	3	0	7
MID-NOON SNACK				
Drink 1.5 to 2 cups of water before meal				
4 oz. raspberries or blue berries and 4 oz. plain organic yogurt (Wait 30 minutes then eat protein snack)	92	6.3	2	12.6
SUPPER				
(Note. drink 1.5 to 2 cups of water)				
8 oz. organic squash or tomato soup	72	2	2	12
4 oz of broiled organic chicken, free range lamb, beef or wild fish				
(Note: use fresh spices like garlic, thyme, parsley)	226	24	14.6	0
12 oz zucchini, kale, spinach, or Swiss chard	40	4.5	0.5	7.5
12 oz. salad with tbsp of olive oil and lemon juice	214	6	20	16
EVENING SNACK				
1 cup herbal tea				
8 oz. organic blueberries, cantaloupe or strawberries chopped	116	3.5	6.5	15.5
(Note. wait half hour to digest the fruit before carb snack)				
4 oz organic oat meal with 8 oz almond milk	120	2	.5	26
TOTALS:	**1866**	**110.3**	**93.45**	**171.7**

Acid Reflux

The medical term for this condition is gastroesophageal reflux disorder (GERD) which may describe conditions such as acid indigestion, Hiatal hernia and reflux esophagitis. One of the main acid reflux occurs when the lower esophageal sphincter (LES), the muscle that connects the esophagus to the upper portion of the stomach does not work properly and allows the partially digested food and hydrochloric acid (HCL) and enzymes back into the esophagus. A second condition is a Hiatal hernia which is when a portion of the stomach is displaced above the diaphragm and the contents of the stomach ends up spilling into the esophagus. Also, diet and lifestyle habits contribute to the GERD condition as well.

Here are some of the main contributors:

- Overeating
- Overweight
- Stress
- Alcohol beverages
- Eating too quickly
- Spicy foods
- Non-steroidal anti-inflammatory drugs like aspirin, ibuprofen and naproxen, bronchodilating drugs for asthma like theophylline, albuterol, ephedrine, blood pressure medications (calcium channel blockers, beta blockers), Valium,

Demerol, nitroglycerine. These medications relax all muscles in the body, including the LES in the esophagus.

- Medications that irritate the intestinal lining are antibiotic tetracycline, anti-arrhythmic drug quinidine, potassium chloride tablets and iron salts
- Fatty and fried foods
- White sugar
- Smoking
- Lying down after eating
- Bending from the waist, heavy lifting and pregnancy which can increase abdominal pressure that can cause GERD
- Not enough chewing
- Caffeine-containing beverages
- Carbonated beverages
- Clothing that constricts the abdomen
- Dehydration
- Tomato based foods, citrus fruits, raw onions, garlic, black pepper, and vinegar
- Ulcers
- Food allergies (especially dairy foods)
- Poor food combining
- Gallbladder problems
- Enzyme deficiencies

Even though the medical profession treats acid indigestion or reflux by using drugs to suppress or neutralize the HCL production, the majority of this condition is caused by not enough HCL or stomach acid.[111] One of the best first lines of treatment is to eat lots of vegetables, organic foods, and fermented foods like sauerkraut, kimchi, fermented cabbage juice, and Himalayan salt. The Himalayan salt has chloride that the body needs to make hydrochloric acid (HCL). The fermented cabbage juice like sauerkraut juice stimulates the body to produce more stomach acid. Furthermore you should be taking one to two probiotic capsules on a daily

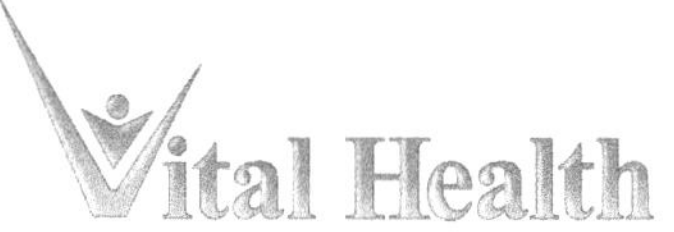

basis as well. Also, a tbsp of raw, unfiltered apple cider vinegar improves the acid content of your stomach. In addition, drinking a half cup of aloe vera juice before each meal reduces inflammation significantly during acid reflux symptoms. Ginger also has gastroprotective properties which block acid. Cut two to three slices of ginger into two cups of hot water and steep for about 30 minutes, then drink it for about 20 minutes before a meal. Finally, Slippery elm tea has amazing affects on acidic conditions. It coats the lining of the mouth, throat, stomach and the intestines and even soothes it from the inflammatory affects of the acid. The following meal plan will have many of the right foods to counter this condition.[112]

STOMACH GASTRITIS

This condition is inflammation of the lining of the stomach where the uppermost mucosal layer starts to erode. This exposes the underlying stomach tissue which is damaged by the enzymes and the hydrochloric acid (HCL). It usually only involves the stomach lining and not the entire stomach wall. It is not an ulcer but an acute or chronic inflammation.

Research has shown that Helicobacter pylori grows exclusively in the mucus secreting cells of the stomach lining and is one of the main causes of chronic gastritis. Only 10 to 15 percent of people with this infection develop gastritis or ulcers. But in underdeveloped countries where sanitation and hygiene are poor, 90 percent are infected. In the U.S., almost two million visits to the doctor of gastritis cases occur per year. Even though this condition occurs in people of all ages and backgrounds, it is especially common in people over 60 years of age, people who drink alcohol excessively, and people who smoke.

Another cause of Gastritis is the use of medicine and non-steroidal anti-inflammatory drugs (NSAIDs) that irritate the stomach lining.[113] Also, chemicals and corrosive compounds that are accidentally swallowed, heavy consumption of strong spices and tobacco can all contribute to this condition. Furthermore, "acute stress gastritis" can occur due to illness or injury such as serious burns or extreme bleeding, high fever, heart attack, and kidney failure. There is also "atrophic gastritis" which is caused by antibodies attacking the stomach lining resulting in the thinning of the lining and loss of acid-producing and enzyme producing cells.[114]

The usual symptoms that appear are the following:

- Heartburn
- Pain in the upper abdomen
- Bloating
- Nausea/vomiting
- Belching
- Black stools (sign of GI bleeding)
- Loss of appetite
- Weight-loss

The standard medical treatment is antibiotics and acid suppressing drugs that protect the stomach lining from being dissolved by the acid and pepsin. However, studies by holistic medical doctor Jonathan Wright have shown that gastritis will actually increase when people infected with the H. pylori take acid suppressing drugs.[115]

Here is the nutritional approach that will greatly help in soothing and improving the stomach lining condition of Gastritis. First of all you should eliminate lifestyle factors that contribute to the condition like regular use of non-steroidal anti-inflammatory drugs (NSAIDs), regular intake of alcohol and smoking. Also make sure you are assessing your condition correctly and not confusing it with other microbial infection, Candida, H. pylori infection or food sensitivity.

Avoid foods such as these that cause irritations with the condition:

- Pepper
- Curry powder
- Cocoa
- Chili

 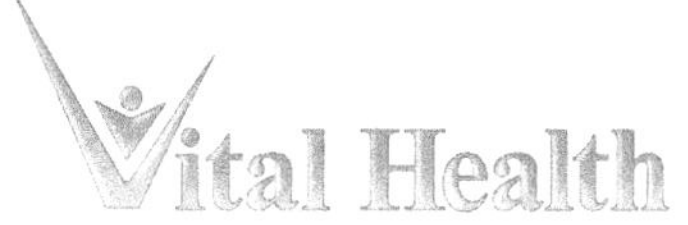

- Chocolate
- Caffeine-containing beverages
- Decaffeinated and regular coffee
- Sugar-containing and processed foods in general

Here are the supplements that can be used to soothe and greatly improve this condition:

- Drink a cup of slippery elm or ginger tea
- Take digestive enzymes that have amylase, lipase and at least 20,000 H.U.T of protease in each capsule, before and after every meal (also the supplement should include marshmallow, ginger, papaya, bromelain, gamma oryzanol and N-acetyl-glucomsamine)
- Chew on one to two 400 mg tablets of deglycyrrhizinated licorice about 20 minutes before meals
- Drink half a cup of aloe vera juice between meals every day
- Take 5,000 to 10,000 mg of glutamine powder with N-acetyl-glucosamine (NAG) and gamma oryzanol once to twice per day on a empty stomach
- Take an ounce of Daily Complete a liquid vitamin/mineral every day
- Take also minimum 3000 mg vitamin C, 10,000 i.u. Vitamin A, 400-800 i.u. Vitamin E, 30-60 mg zinc,
- Take three to six 1000 mg of omega-3 fish and flax oils and omega-6 borage oil in capsules twice daily with food
- Take a probiotic capsule with minimum of 2 to 6 billion cultures every day
- Take a B-12 vitamin every day
- Take a Folic acid supplement every day
- Take a liquid iron supplement by Flora called Floradix, order on their website: requiredforlife.com (Take only if iron and ferritin levels are low)

Furthermore, sleeping on your left side helps with the indigestion. Do not lie down at least for 3-4 hours after eating. Also, elevate your head on the pillow in bed about 4-8 inches when sleeping.[116]

Peptic Ulcers

An ulcer is a sore or lesion that develops in the mucus lining of the stomach, duodenum and the esophagus. The reason it's called a peptic ulcer is the lesion or sore in the lining of these organs exposes it to the stomach acids and pepsin which is the protein-digesting enzyme produced in the stomach. Duodenal ulcer is the most common and occurs four to five times more than stomach ulcers. Esophageal ulcers are rare. They can however, develop from acid reflux.

It used to be that stress was considered as the main factor, but studies have shown that this is not the case. What seems to be one of the main causes is the presence of the bacterium, Helicobacter pylori (H. pylori) in between the lining of the stomach and the protective mucous layer. Researchers are not sure how people contract this bacterium, but it is believed that it is contracted through food, water or mouth-to-mouth contact. It weakens the mucous lining gradually leaving it exposed to the acids of the stomach. Also H. pylori is not the only cause, but quite a few other factors seem to be the cause.

Here is the list of the various contributors:

- Regular use of NSAIDs
- Use of steroid drugs like cortisone
- Alcohol consumption (moderate to excessive)
- Heavy smoking

- A family history of peptic ulcer disease
- Stress
- Nutritional deficiencies
- A low-fibre diet
- Food allergies
- Caffeine-containing beverages
- Dehydration
- Severe illness or trauma (causing a "stress ulcer")

One factor that I want to go over is the importance of drinking water to help this condition. Studies done by Dr. Batmanghelidj found that the stomach needs lots of water to produce enough mucus.[117] Over 25-million Americans develop peptic ulcer at some point in their lives.[118]You usually experience gastric pain and irritation when the stomach is empty, so when you eat, the food acts as a buffer where it neutralizes the acid which relieves the pain of duodenal ulcers. The symptoms of peptic ulcers are:

- Headache
- A choking sensation
- Nausea/vomiting
- Back pain
- Black tarry stools
- Paleness
- Weakness
- Loss of appetite
- Weight loss
- Dizziness

The normal medical treatment is antibiotics and acid-suppressing drugs. There are two steps that can be followed from a nutritional approach. Step one is to first eradicate the H. pylori and step two is through supplementing with natural herbs, vitamins and wholesome foods.

Step One:

- 250 mg Mastic gum four times a day
- 3000 mg vitamin C powder per day

- 240 mg of Bismuth subcitrate twice a day available from compounding pharmacies
- Use anti-fungal and anti-bacterial such as grapefruit seed extract, garlic, rosemary,[119] thyme extracts in tincture form every day [120]
- Take probiotics every day

Step Two:

- Step two is using supplements that will greatly help in soothing and improving the stomach lining condition of Peptic Ulcers:
- Chew on one to two 400 mg tablets of deglycyrrhizinated licorice about 20 minutes before meals [121]
- Half cup of aloe vera juice between meals [122]
- 5000 to 20,000 mg of Glutamine powder with gamma oryzanol daily on a empty stomach
- Some ginger, calendula and cranesbill herbs in tincture form every day
- Take a probiotic capsule with minimum of 2 to 6 billion cultures every day
- Take also minimum 3000 mg vitamin C, 10,000 i.u. vitamin A, 400-800 i.u. vitamin E, 30-60 mg zinc,
- Take three to six 1000 mg of omega-3 fish and flax oils and omega-6 borage oil in capsules twice daily with food
- Take one 30 g scoop of a natural fibre supplement that provides a balance of both soluble and insoluble fibres like a flax and borage seed mixture
- Take a liquid iron supplement by Flora called Floradix on their website: requiredforlife.com (Take only if iron and ferritin levels are low

The meal plan given in the following page is for Gastritis, Peptic Ulcers and Acid Reflux. It can be followed as an example of the foods that you should stick to as much as possible when you are struggling with these conditions. You will notice I always put in a glass of fresh vegetable juice recipe in the meal plans. The reason for this is it is full of concentrated nutrition without the fibre, so the digestive system does not have to work too hard and helps in allowing the alkaline balance of the gut to be restored.[123]

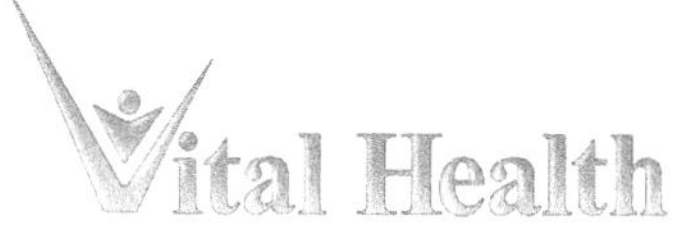

ACID INDIGESTION, GASTRITIS AND PEPTIC ULCER MEAL PLAN

UPON WAKING	CAL.	PROTEIN(G)	FAT(G)	CARBS.(G)
Drink 3 to 6 glasses of water upon the first hour and half of waking up (Note. 8 glasses of water if wrong combination of foods eaten the day before) Also add 1 tbsp organic unfiltered apple cider vinegar in a glass of water and drink it down				
4-8 oz fresh organic raspberries, blueberries with sprinkle of cinnamon with 8 oz. unsweetened almond milk.	100	1.7	3.5	16
(Note. wait half hour to digest the fruit before breakfast; also drink half glass of aloe vera juice which helps reduce inflammation during acid indigestion flare-ups) 1 tbsp omega-3 oil or 3 capsules of fish oil, one powdered capsule of 50 mg vitamin B complex, 1 tsp Vitamin C powder, and 1 capsule of probiotic supplement which has more than a billion good bacteria in it. 2 level tbsp of liquid Daily Complete	130	0	13.5	0
BREAKFAST A Note. you have the option of only having breakfast A or B in the mornings, hence your calorie total for the day will be less; however you can have both on days you are hungry)				
(Note. I suggest not to use milk with cereal but if you really find it hard to change, please at least get organic milk)				
8 oz. organic unsweetened almond or rice milk	40	1	3.5	2
4 oz. seed cereal with 2-3 tbsp of flax seeds added	65	1	1	11.5
8-12 oz. veg. / fruit. Juice (8 oz. spinach or cabbage, carrots and 4 inch chunk ginger)	69	1.9	0.35	16.1
BREAKFAST B 12 oz of salad of sliced cucumbers, green pepper, fennel, parsley, oregano, mint, spinach or cabbage, two crushed garlic clove and ½ inch slice Spanish onion	50	3	0	7
1 tbsp olive oil & squeezed lemon juice	119		14	
2 free range eggs (poached, boiled or scrambled)	160	12	10	1
1 cup Slippery elm tea	7	1	0	1

MID-MORNING SNACK (OPTIONAL IF HUNGRY) 1 c of Pure Trim shake	86	14.6	1.3	4
(Note. Recipe for 3 cup protein shake: 2.5 cups of water, 1 banana, 4 oz. fresh or frozen strawberries, ½ pack Pure Trim and 1-2 oz. unsweetened almond milk or goat's milk)				
LUNCH (Note. drink 1.5 to 2 cups of water)				
Drink ½ cup of water mixed with ½ of cup of raw potato juice with skin left on made in a juicer [124]	292	8		67
4 oz. organic wild salmon, mackerel, or haddock baked, broiled or BBQ	208	30.6	8	0
12 oz. broccoli, Brussell sprouts, green beans, kale, or cauliflower, etc., with a ½ tsp of Himalayan sea salt, ground pepper	40	4.5	0.5	7.5
MID-NOON SNACK Drink 1 cup of water and 1 cup cabbage juice before mid-noon meal or snack				
4-8 oz raspberries, blue berries (Note. wait 30 minutes then eat protein snack)	60	.7		14
4 oz low fat organic plain yogurt with tsp maple syrup	85	6	2	11.5
SUPPER (Note. drink 1.5 to 2 cups of water)				
4 oz of organic chicken, free range beef , lamb or wild fish broiled, baked or steamed	226	24	14.6	0
8 oz. broccoli, Brussell sprouts, kale, or cauliflower, etc., with a ½ tsp of Himalayan sea salt & pepper	40	4.5	0.5	7.5
12 oz. salad with 1 tbsp olive oil & lemon juice and 4 oz of sauerkraut with tsp of organic salad dressing	122	6	21	20
EVENING SNACK 1 cup Ginger tea				
4oz. fresh raspberries, blue berries and black berries (Note. Wait 30 minutes before eating the crackers)	20	0.3	Trace	4.6
13 five Mary's Organic crackers (gluten free)	140	3	5	21
TOTALS:	**2059**	**123.8**	**98.75**	**211.7**

Accelerated Weight Loss or Lean Up

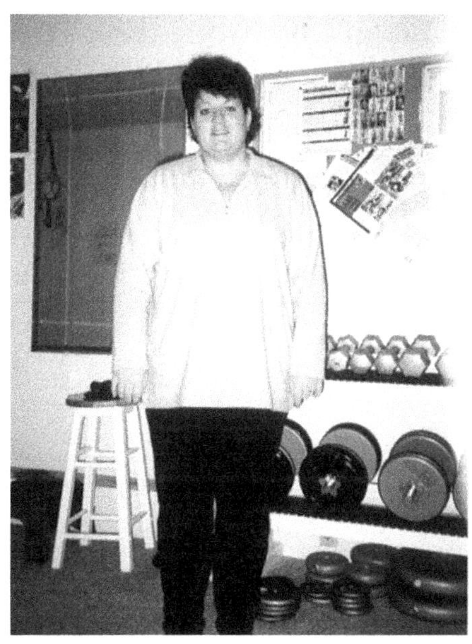

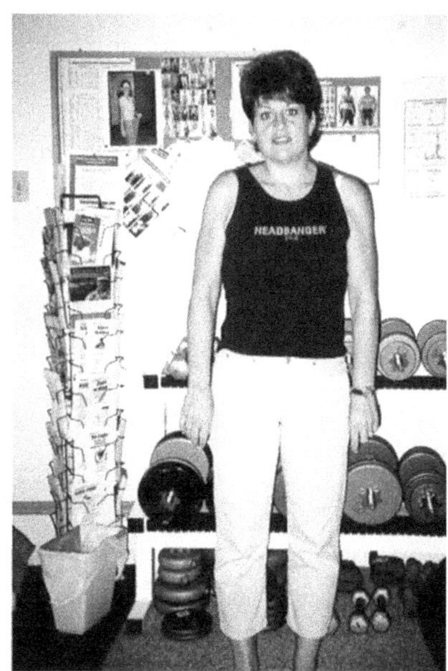

I know weight-loss is a "huge" concern with many people even though most people suppress their deep feelings of discouragement over their inability to overcome this challenge. I'm here to tell you that it can be overcome. Here is one of several pictures of some of my clients in the past who have lost weight and are keeping it off. This client lost over 100 pounds using the Vital Health System of nutrition and exercise.

I am going to be very direct and truthful about this issue. It is discipline and self-control on how much you eat of any given food that has a lot to do with gaining excess fat and weight. There is nothing wrong with treating yourself with a sugary dessert or a bacon sandwich once in awhile. Your body can handle digesting this heavy treat as long as the other 90 percent of the time you are eating healthy and balanced meals. These healthy meals are loaded with high amount of nutrients, anti-oxidants, fibre, vitamins, minerals and enzymes. I personally eat according to this type of approach. However, I have come to the point where even my treats still need to contain a good amount of nutritional value in them. For example, when I feel like a good dessert I go to a local vegetarian restaurant called The Green Door. They make their pies and cakes from spelt, organic grain, low gluten or gluten-free, organic fruits and natural sweeteners like maple syrup and unpasteurized honey. My system still feels good after eating their desserts, main courses and breads. It's because the nutrient content of the foods is very high compared to the foods you eat at an average restaurant. You will find that as you become healthier and more fit, your body will be more in tune to what foods are agreeable with your system and which ones are not. I cannot really eat desserts or meals that have processed ingredients, refined flour and refined sugar without my stomach reacting in some way to the sudden pollution. It just does not feel good! I feel bloated, full of gas and lethargic. My tight, flat stomach and waistline feels like it's added another inch.

Another factor you need to consider is the idea of regular exercise for about an hour, three to five times a week. It should be a combination of some floor body exercises, stretching, some resistance with weights and some form of cardio activity. This allows you to burn any excess calories and fat so you stay trim, not to mention the firmness and tone your muscles will have on a consistent basis. Let's face it, when your body feels like this you "feel like a million bucks"! The quality of your life is greatly improved and not to mention the self-image and social confidence!

Even though I don't believe you need to count every calorie when you are trying to lose excess fat and weight, you still need to know roughly the total amount of calories you need in order for your body to carry out its normal functions, to carry out your physical movements outside of exercise and to carry out your workout. My plans here are to get you to retain and increase your lean muscle and decrease your fat percentage. The weight number you see on the scale is not as important as the body composition that you have. Also my weight-loss program should be combined with some sort of physical exercise program to give you the best results.

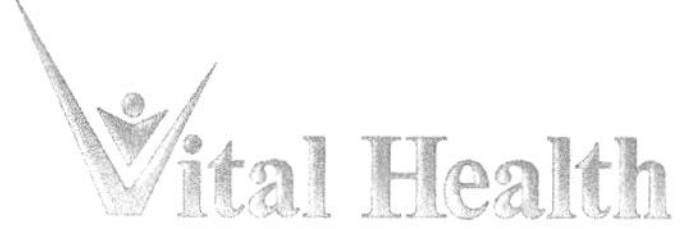

Your body was made to move, stretch, climb, walk and run. If you are carrying more than 20 pounds of body weight and have not been doing any exercises for a long time, then start with light aerobic activity like power-walking outside or on the treadmill, bicycling, stair climbing, swimming or moving on a cross trainer for 30 minutes every day with about 30 minutes of floor work focusing on core, calisthenics and stretching. This will increase your metabolic rate so that you are burning more calories even when resting. Another option is you may want to get my Vital Health exercise videos which are available on my website. They will show you how to carry out basic floor exercises to get your whole body in shape, more flexible and stronger.

ACCELERATED WEIGHT-LOSS

Studies have shown that lowering calories and increasing your exercise is the safest and most effective way to lose weight. I have provided two kinds of calculations to estimate your calorie total for best results. For those who need to lose a significant amount of weight, over 20 pounds, you can use the calculations under Accelerated Weight-loss Formula. In addition, the meal plan for the Accelerated Weight-loss is given on the next few pages. Depending on how active you are in your lifestyle or how intense your workouts are, you may have to adjust your calorie intake by increasing or decreasing by 200-300 calories or more. I suggest you take in the extra calories in the form of raw nuts, nut bar, extra Pure Trim protein shake or replace a snack with a small meal of salad mixed with pieces of chicken, beef or fish. Metabolic rates are hard to establish so you may have to play around with this adjustment at the beginning until you find the best balance of fuel intake.[125]

ACCELERATED WEIGHT-LOSS FORMULA

Here you can calculate what you want your ideal weight to be, then you can calculate the total calories you need to eat per day to start losing weight. The formula consists of you putting in the ideal weight you want to be, and then use the following calculations:

(Female) Your Ideal Weight: ______ x 3.95 + 825 calories = Your Caloric Limit for the day

(Male) Your Ideal Weight: ______ x 5.3 + 879 calories = Your Caloric Limit for the day [126]

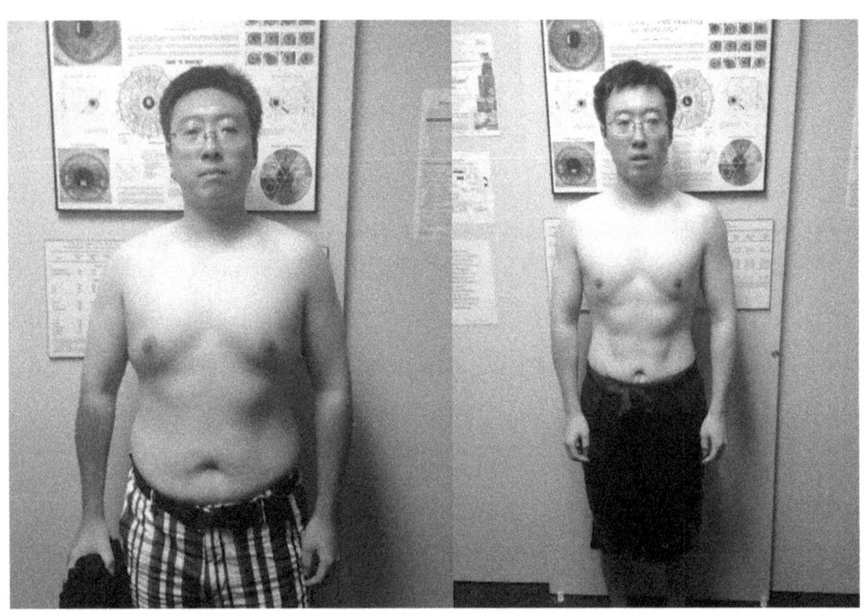

LEAN UP

For those who only need to lose five to 15 pounds of extra fat, are working out quite seriously and are quite advanced in their training abilities with a pretty intense cardio program, you should follow the calculations under the Lean Up Formula. My male client in these pictures was training for a few years, but was not getting results, even with the help of trainers. This is where the proper nutrition can make such a huge difference. Also, I have provided a sample meal plan for one week of the meals and snacks that could work to help fuel your body and lean you up at the same time in the One Week Lean Up Plan. In addition, I have put together pages of recipes that you can use in this meal plan following the page of the One Week Lean Up Plan.

To calculate the calorie needs you have to keep your body functions going is called your resting metabolic rate (RMR). This is calculated by multiplying your bodyweight by 10. So if you weigh 160 Ibs, your RMR would be 1600 calories. Also to calculate your calorie needs outside of exercise, multiply your RMR amount by 20%. Therefore, in this case, the daily activity burn is 320 calories. Furthermore, add 600 calories needed for the exercise period and you have your total calorie required for the day which would be 2520 calories.[127]

LEAN UP FORMULA

RMR Calculation: Your Body Weight X 10 = RMR (Resting Metabolic Rate)
Daily Activity Burn Calculation: Your RMR X 20% = DAB (Daily Activity Burn)
Total Energy Burn: Your RMR + Your DAB + 600 = TEB (Total Energy Burn)
1600 + 320 + 600 = 2520 Calories

You will notice that most of the sample meal plans in the One Week Lean Up Plan are around 2500 calories. Again there are always exceptions to the rule. If you are a male or female athlete then you may need significantly more calories. If you are heavy boned and a bigger framed female like some of the female athletes in sports like rugby, shot putting, power-lifting, and bodybuilding then your calorie needs may be higher. If you are a track athlete who sprints and does any of the distance runs on the track like the 1500 meter race, then because of the high output of calories burned in such sports, even though your weight may be light as a female or male runner, your total calorie needs may be much higher than normal.

However, for most people, the calorie total that I have put together here for both weight-loss categories seems to work. Even if you are not an athlete in training, you should monitor how you feel when you are following either one of the weight-loss plans. If you feel you need to eat more on some days because you had higher amounts of activity such as a longer run, a high impact aerobic class or a kickboxing class, you should increase your protein intake in the plan by twice the amount and also add a 4 to 8 ounce of complex carb like steamed or baked sweet potato, brown rice or rice pasta as an extra meal on that day.

As mentioned earlier, any of the recipes under The Accelerated Weight-Loss and Lean Recipes can be used in any of the meals outlined in the Accelerated Weight-Loss sheet or the One Week Lean Up Plan sheet. Some of the meal recipes are not properly combined. Also try to get unsweetened almond milk for the days where the plan specifies you drink almond milk or skim milk. You do have protein with some complex carbohydrates like wild rice and grain bagel. You can cheat and ignore the food combining for two to three meals per week. I find the body can handle it, as long as you are drinking enough water, taking in some raw fresh vegetable juice, and some probiotic supplements. Also consume lots of raw vegetable salads with each meal and take the cleansing product Experience in the evening.

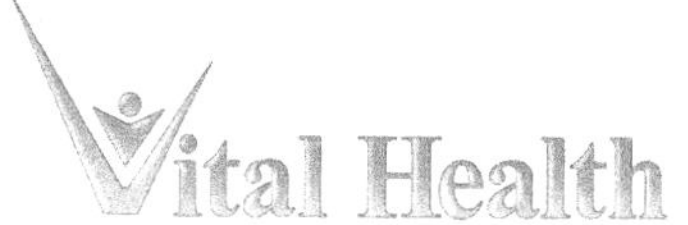

ACCELERATED WEIGHT LOSS MEAL PLAN

UPON WAKING	CAL.	PROTEIN(G)	FAT(G)	CARB(G)
Drink 3 to 6 glasses of water upon the first hour and half of waking up (Note. 8 glasses of water if wrong combination of foods eaten the day before)				
Go for a 30-45 minute power-walk preferably in outdoors, then 15-30 minutes core, floor work and stretches				
After shower apply Pure Gardens Cream on face and body (Note. this helps tighten skin and wrinkles, if interested go to retail site: vitalcleanse.puretrim.com)				
BREAKFAST				
1 tbsp omega-3 oil or 3 capsules of fish oil, one powder capsule 50 mg. vitamin B complex, 1 level tsp Vitamin C powder (about 1500 mg) 2 level tbsp of liquid Daily Complete	130	0	13.5	0
8 oz fruits i.e. banana, apple, nectarine, berries, etc.	50	0.5	Trace	26
(Note. wait half hour to digest the fruit before the shake)				
Have a 12 oz Pure Trim Shake then 2 full glasses of water right after	86	14.6	1.3	4
(Note. 3 cup Pure Trim recipe: 2.5 cups of water, 1 or ½ banana, 4-6 oz fresh fruit or frozen fruit,1 pack Pure Trim shake ; 1-2 oz unsweetened almond milk if desired)				
MID-MORNING (OPTIONAL)				
(if hungry have 1-2 eggs (poached, boiled or scrambled) or 2-4 oz tuna or chicken with 4 oz sliced cucumbers, celery and tomatoes	160	12	12	0
LUNCH				
(Note. drink 1.5 to 2 cups of water)				
Drink 1.5 to 2 cups of water before meal				
4-6 oz chicken, seafood, turkey, beef, lean lamb				
(with spices, garlic and 2 oz of meat juices)	464	46	30	0
8-12 oz broccoli, Brussell sprouts, green beans, kale, cauliflower, etc., with a ½ tsp of sea salt, ground pepper	40	4.5	0.5	7.5
8- 12 oz salad 1 tbsp organic salad dressing				
(Note. No Dairy or Gluten foods)	67	0	6.5	7

MID-NOON SNACK Drink 1.5 to 2 cups of water before snack				
4-8 oz pineapple or other fruits (Note. wait 30 minutes then eat protein snack)	50	.5		26
½ oz raw almonds	78	2.5	6.7	3
SUPPER (Note. drink 1.5 to 2 cups of water)				
Have a 12 oz Pure Trim Shake (Note. then 2 full glasses of water right after)	86	14.6	1.3	4
EVENING SNACK				
1 cup herbal tea				
4-8 oz pineapple or other fruits	50	.5		26
½oz raw almonds	78	2.5	6.7	3
Take Experience (cleansing product) as you have a quiet time, read, movie				
Apply Pure Gardens Serum on face and body (optional)				
Go to bed by 10:30pm				
TOTAL:	**1339**	**98.2**	**78.5**	**106.5**

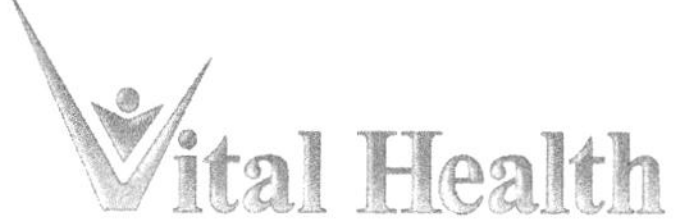

ONE WEEK SAMPLE LEAN UP PLAN

	BREAKFAST	SNACK	LUNCH	SNACK	DINNER
DAY 1	1 cup fresh strawberries (Note. eat 30 min before meal) 1 Mushroom Omelet, 8 oz of 1% or low fat cottage cheese or ricotta cheese	1 Protein Bar or Nut Bar and Protein Shake	Bowl of Vital Health Salad	1 oz unsalted roasted or raw almonds	6 oz Linda's Battered Wild Salmon Steaks ½cup asparagus steamed, 1 cup wild rice, 1 cup vegetable soup, (if desired, add1 tbsp non-flavoured protein powder to soup before serving)
DAY 2	1 Protein Shake	1 Protein Bar or Nut Bar and Protein Shake	Shrimp Stir-Fry, 1 tbsp sesame seeds, 1 oz cashews	1- ½oz low fat cheese	6 oz Roasted Organic Chicken, 2 tbsp gravy, ½ cup green beans, 1 cup butternut squash soup or vegetable soup of your choice (boxed organic, found at health food stores) 1 tbsp non-flavored protein powder
DAY 3	4 oz fresh squeezed juice of your choice, or done in a juicer (Note. have 30 min before meal) 2 Slices fresh preservative free chicken or smoked turkey cold cut (Nitrate free), 1 Chicken Scramble	1 Protein Bar or Nut Bar and Protein Shake	1 Chicken Salad & 2 cups salad greens, 1 cup vegetable soup, add 1 tbsp non-flavoured protein powder	1 oz unsalted roasted or raw almonds	6 oz Halibut, cod, red snapper or haddock, 2 tbsp pesto sauce, 1 cup wild rice, ½cup zucchini steamed

DAY 4	organic chicken, turkey or lean beef sausage on whole grain bagel & 8 oz skim milk, or almond milk	1 Protein Bar or Nut Bar and Protein Shake	1 Steak and green salad, 2 tbsp balsamic vinaigrette dressing	1 oz natural preservative free Beef Jerky	6 oz Chicken breast, 2 tbsp honey-chili sauce, 1 cup quinoa, ½cup snap peas
DAY 5	½grapefruit (Note. have 30 min before meal) 1 Spinach scramble, & 8 oz skim milk, or almond milk	1 Protein Bar or Nut Bar and Protein Shake	6 oz Turkey burger, ½oz low fat Swiss cheese, ½cup coleslaw, 1 cup organic tomato, butternut squash soup, 1 tbsp non-flavored protein powder	4 oz strawberries, blueberries, or cantaloupe(Note. have 30 min before meal) 8 oz low fat ricotta cheese	6 oz mackerel, halibut, haddock or cod, 2 tbsp mango-ginger sauce, 1 cup wild rice steamed, 1 artichoke (canned or fresh)
DAY 6	1 Protein Shake	1 Protein Bar or Nut Bar and Protein Shake	1 chicken salad	1 oz natural preservative free Beef Jerky	1 Beef & broccoli stir-fry, 1 cup miso soup, 1 tbsp non-flavored protein powder
DAY 7	1/4 cantaloupe (Note. have 30 min before meal) 2 slices fresh preservative free chicken or smoked turkey cold cut (Nitrate free), 1 cheese scramble, 8 oz skim milk or almond milk	1 Protein Bar or Nut Bar and Protein Shake	1 Tuna salad, 2 oz Vital Health Wakame Seaweed Salad, 1 cup squash soup or tomato soup of your choice (Note. boxed organic, found at health food stores)	4 oz strawberries, blueberries, or cantaloupe (Note. have 30 min before) 8 oz low fat ricotta cheese	6 oz Lemon-garlic chicken, 1 cup wild rice, 1 cup squash soup or tomato soup of your choice (boxed organic, found at health food stores), 1 tbsp non-flavored protein powder

Accelerated Weight Loss and Lean Up Recipes

PER SERVING
191 Calories
5 g Total Fat
38 g Protein
7 g Carbohydrate
596 mg Sodium

MUSHROOM OMELET (2 SERVINGS)

6 oz egg whites (1 egg = 1 oz egg white)
Sea salt & pepper to taste
3/4 cup Shitake mushrooms sliced
3 tbsp Spanish onion chopped
½ tomato chopped
1 ounce low-fat Mozzarella cheese shredded

In a small bowl, lightly beat the egg whites with a fork and season to taste with pinch of garlic powder, sea salt and pepper. Coat the non-stick pan with 1 tbsp cold pressed olive oil and place over medium heat (Note. use a non-Teflon coated pan as much as possible because of the possible toxic effects of the Teflon [128]). Add the vegetables and cook until tender. Add egg mixture and cook until set on the bottom. Sprinkle the cheese over top, fold omelet in half after cheese is melted and eggs are set.

CHICKEN SCRAMBLE (2 SERVINGS)

8 oz egg white with 1 whole egg
3 ounces chicken breast, cooked and diced
2 tbsp skim milk, almond milk
1 ounces part-skim mozzarella cheese grated
1 tbsp chopped fresh basil

PER SERVING

439 Calories
14.6 g Total Fat
52.6 g Protein
4 g Carbohydrate
312 mg Cholesterol
376 mg Sodium

Coat a small non-stick pan with 1 tbsp cold pressed olive oil and place over medium heat. In a small bowl, lightly beat the egg whites and egg with a fork and add to the pan. Cook, stir, until halfway set, then add the diced chicken and cook through. Add pinch of sea salt and pepper to taste. Garnish with fresh basil and serve.

ORGANIC TURKEY SAUSAGE ON WHOLE GRAIN BAGEL (1 SERVING)

4 ounces organic smoked turkey sausage
1 whole grain bagel
1 oz of low fat mozzarella cheese
Three thin slices of tomato
Four thin slices of cucumber

PER SERVING

444 Calories
15 g Total Fat
30.6 g Protein
46.3 g Carbohydrate
76.6 mg Cholesterol
1102 mg Sodium

Slice your bagel into two pieces and slice your sausage in half length wise, then cut it in half. Place the sausage pieces on one bagel half. Then place the piece of cheese on top. Top with slices of cucumber and tomato and put it in the toaster oven for about 3-5 minutes until cheese melts and the bagel gets nice and toasted.

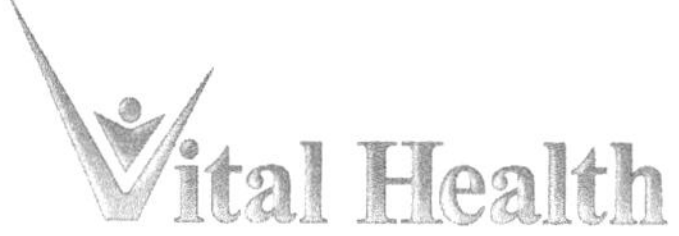

SPINACH SCRAMBLE (2 SERVINGS)

½ cup tomato, diced
1 cup organic Spinach leaves, cleaned and dried
6 oz egg white with 1 whole egg added
½ oz feta cheese, crumbled
1 tbsp fresh basil chopped

PER SERVING
292 Calories
13 g Total Fat
33 g Protein
232 g Cholesterol
10 g Carbohydrate
835 mg Sodium

Coat a small non-stick pan with 1 tbsp cold pressed olive oil, sauté tomatoes and spinach until slightly tender. Remove and set aside. Whisk the egg whites and egg together in a bowl and add to the pan. Cook, stirring, over low heat until almost set. Add the vegetable mixture, cheese, and basil. Cook to desired firmness.

CHEF SALAD (1 SERVING)

3 ounces of cooked turkey or chicken breast, chopped
3 ounces of preservative free smoked turkey (Nitrate free)
1 oz of low fat mozzarella cheese, chopped
½ tomato, chopped
2 cups romaine lettuce, chopped
½ cup of sliced cucumbers
1/4 cup of diced green, red pepper
1 ounce of avocado diced (optional)
2 tbsp organic salad dressing

PER SERVING
371 calories
12.6 g Total Fat
50 g Protein
14 g Carbohydrate
102 mg Cholesterol
515 mg Sodium

Toss ingredients together in a bowl and drizzle with dressing.

SHRIMP STIR FRY (2 SERVINGS)

6 ounces large shrimp, peeled
½ tbsp low -sodium tamari sauce
1 tsp rice vinegar
½ cup chicken broth
½ tsp garlic and ginger minced
1 cup red or Spanish onion sliced in wedges
1 cup organic broccoli florets
1 cup snow peas trimmed
1 cup Shitake mushrooms in quarters
½ cup organic yellow or red bell pepper, cubed
½ cup canned water chestnuts, drained (optional)

PER SERVING
332 calories
4 g Total Fat
44 g Protein
33 g Carbohydrate
259 mg Cholesterol
552 mg Sodium

Rinse shrimp and drain well. Heat the tamari sauce, rice vinegar, and 2 tbsp of the chicken broth *(use MSG-free chicken soup base powder)* in a sauté pan over medium heat. Add the garlic and ginger and sauté until tender. Add all the vegetables to the pan and continue to sauté, stirring and adding more broth as necessary. Add shrimp when the vegetables are halfway cooked and sauté until the vegetables are tender and the shrimp are opaque.

CHICKEN SALAD (2 SERVINGS)

8 ounces boneless, skinless chicken breast halves
2 tbsp low fat mayonnaise
1 tbsp Dijon mustard
2 tbsp green onions diced
1/4 tsp black pepper
½ cup organic celery diced
1/4 tsp fresh dill

PER SERVING
345 Calories
12 g Total Fat
43 g Protein
14 g Carbohydrate
105 mg Cholesterol
361 mg Sodium

Poach chicken (boil in water): cool and dice. Gently combine the chicken with the remaining ingredients and chill until ready to serve.

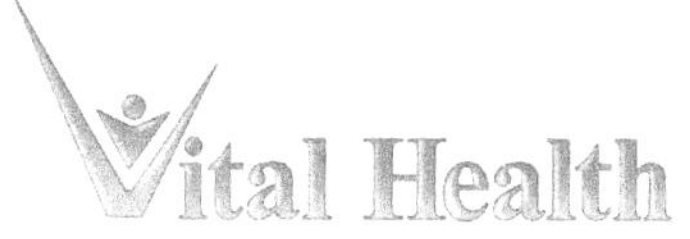

STEAK AND GREEN SALAD (2 SERVINGS)

8 ounces of top sirloin
3 cups of spinach, romaine or endive, leaves
½ pint cherry tomatoes, halved
3/4 cup canned artichoke hearts, drained
3 tbsp of balsamic vinaigrette dressing

PER SERVING
531 Calories
14 g Total Fat
51 g Protein
26 g Carbohydrate
116 mg Cholesterol
414 mg Sodium

Grill, barbeque or broil steak until done, approximately 7 to 10 minutes on each side. Cool and cut into 1-inch slices. Toss together the green lettuce leaves, tomatoes and artichoke hearts and arrange on plate. Top with the steak and drizzle with balsamic vinaigrette.

TURKEY BURGER (2 SERVINGS)

8 ounces of ground turkey breast
1-2 tbsp of organic bread crumbs
6 tbsp low-fat butter milk
4- ½ tsp of green onion, minced
4- ½ tsp parsley, chopped
½ tsp Dijon mustard
2 dashes Worcestershire sauce, black pepper to taste.

PER SERVING
410 Calories
16 g Total Fat
49 g Protein
14 g Carbohydrate
135 mg Cholesterol
351 mg Sodium

Preheat the grill or broiler. Combine all ingredients and form into patty, Grill until cooked through, 7-10 minutes per side.

TUNA SALAD (2 SERVINGS)

8 ounces tuna, canned in water
1 ounce Nutrimax mayonnaise (natural ingredients)
1 tsp lemon juice (freshly squeezed)
1 ounce carrots, shredded
1 ounce organic celery, chopped
1 tbsp green onion, chopped
1 tsp celery seeds (optional)

PER SERVING
337 Calories
11 g Total Fat
59 g Protein
8 g Carbohydrates
68 mg Cholesterol
447 Sodium

Drain canned tuna, place in a bowl. Add mayonnaise and mix thoroughly. Then add lemon juice, carrots, celery, green onions, and celery seeds. Blend together.

LEMON-DILL SAUCE (10 SERVINGS)

½cup Spanish onions, chopped
2 cups of white wine
2 tbsp arrowroot
2 cups of chicken broth (Non-MSG- soup base)
6 tbsp lemon juice
1 tsp lemon grass, minced
1 tbsp fresh dill, chopped

PER SERVING
58 Calories
trace Total Fat
3 g Protein
5 g Carbohydrate
0 mg Cholesterol
107 mg Sodium

Coat a large sauté pan with olive oil spray, or use 1-2 tbsp cold pressed olive oil or sunflower oil and sauté onions until soft (not brown), moistening with wine if necessary.

Dissolve the arrow root in ½ cup of the chicken broth. Set aside. Add remaining wine to onions and reduce heat by half. Add remaining chicken broth and reduce by half again.

Add the arrowroot mixture. Transfer the mixture to a food processor or blender and puree until smooth. Return the sauce to the pan. Add lemon juice and lemongrass and simmer over low heat for about 30 minutes, until thick. Strain out the lemongrass and stir in the dill.

CHILLED CUCUMBER SOUP (4 SERVINGS)

1 Whole cucumber
½cup red onions, chopped
3 tbsp fresh dill, chopped
1 tbsp fresh mint, chopped
1-1/4 cup non-fat plain yogurt
1/4 tsp sea salt

PER SERVING
60 Calories
trace Total Fat
5 g Protein
10 g Carbohydrate
1 mg Cholesterol
191 mg Sodium

Add 1/8 tsp black pepper, 1/16 tsp cayenne pepper, and 1/4 tbsp celery seed. Combine all ingredients and puree with blender. Chill. Garnish with chopped dill or parsley.

BALSAMIC VINAIGRETTE (16 SERVINGS)

1- ½ cups balsamic vinegar
2 tbsp fresh lemon juice
6 tbsp Dijon mustard
4 tsp shallots or onions, chopped
4 tsp fresh basil, chopped
2 tsp olive oil

PER SERVING
14 Calories
1 g Total Fat
0 g Protein
2 g Carbohydrate
0 mg Cholesterol
71 mg Sodium

Add black pepper to taste. Whisk together all ingredients in a small bowl. Store covered in a dressing bottle preferably, in the refrigerator.

VEGETABLE SOUP (18 SERVINGS)

10 cups fat-free chicken broth, low sodium
4 potatoes cut into 1-inch cubes
4 cups onions, quartered
1 cup carrots, sliced 1-inch thick
3 cups celery, sliced 1-inch thick
2 cups zucchini, sliced 1-inch thick
8 ounces tomato sauce, canned.
2 cloves garlic minced,
1/4 bunch fresh parsley chopped
1/4 bunch cilantro chopped, dash black pepper

PER SERVING
49 Calories
trace Total Fat
7 g Protein
10 g Carbohydrate
0 mg Cholesterol
77 mg Sodium

In a large stockpot, combine the chicken broth, potatoes, onions, carrots, and celery. Bring to a boil, reduce heat to medium-high, and simmer until the potatoes are tender for about 30 minutes. Add the zucchini, tomato sauce, garlic, parsley, and cilantro. Reduce heat to medium-low and cook for 10 to 15 minutes more, or until the zucchini is just tender. Season to taste with black pepper and serve. If desired, add 1 scoop of non-flavoured protein powder just before serving.

GRAVY (10 SERVINGS)

1/3 cup shallots or onions, chopped
1/3 cup all almond flour
3 cups fat-free chicken broth, low sodium
1/4 tsp sea salt
1 tsp poultry seasoning

PER SERVING
34 Calories
trace Total Fat
4 g Protein
4 g Carbohydrate
0 mg Cholesterol
229 mg Sodium

Sauté shallots or onions in some of the broth until soft. Gradually whisk in the flour, adding broth as needed to form a thick paste. Gradually add the remaining broth, stirring and cooking until thickened. Add the salt and poultry seasoning.

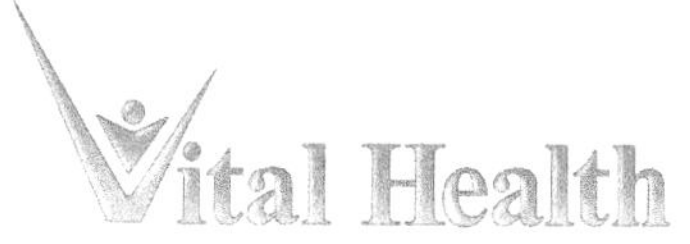

PESTO SAUCE (20 SERVINGS)

1 cup pine nuts
4 cups fresh basil
2 tbsp garlic, chopped
1 cup fat-free parmesan cheese, grated
1/3 cup white cooking wine
1/3 cup lemon juice
½ cup fat-free chicken broth (Non-MSG)
½ tsp sea salt

PER SERVING
61 calories
4 g Total Fat
4 g Protein
4 g Carbohydrate
5 mg Cholesterol
110 mg Sodium

Heat skillet over medium-high heat and toasted pine nuts, turning until golden brown.

In food processor, puree basil, toasted pine nuts and garlic. Add Parmesan cheese, wine, lemon juice, chicken broth and process until blended. Add salt to taste and blend. Serve on pasta, chicken, or seafood.

HONEY-CHILE SAUCE (16 SERVINGS)

1/4 cup shallots or onions, chopped fine
2/3 cup honey, slightly warmed
1/4 cup sherry vinegar or wine vinegar
1 tsp chili powder
1/4 tsp ground cumin
1- ½ cups fat-free chicken broth (Non-MSG)
Sea salt and pepper to taste
1 tsp cilantro, chopped
3 tbsp chopped pecans, toasted

PER SERVING
56 Calories
1 g Total Fat
1 g Protein
13 g Carbohydrate
0 mg Cholesterol
48 mg Sodium

Coat a pan with olive oil cooking spray, or use 1-2 tbsp cold pressed safflower oil and place on medium high heat. Add chopped shallots or onions and sauté until tender. Add the honey and vinegar to the pan. Quickly stir in the chili powder, cumin, and broth. Bring to a boil and reduce by half the heat. Transfer sauce to a blender or food processor and blend at a high speed until smooth. Season to taste with sea salt and pepper. Stir in cilantro. Garnish dish with toasted pecans.

MANGO-GINGER SAUCE (8 SERVINGS)

½ tbsp olive oil
1 cup red onion, finely chopped
1 cup mango, peeled and cubed
½cup tomato, chopped
1- ½ tbsp fresh ginger, minced
1/4 cup fresh lime juice
2 tbsp orange juice
2 tbsp dry sherry
1- ½ tbsp brown sugar
1- ½ tbsp white vinegar

PER SERVING
46 Calories
1 g Total Fat
1 g Protein
9 g Carbohydrate
0 mg Cholesterol
3 mg Sodium

Stir together all ingredients in a nonreactive bowl. Store covered in the refrigerator until ready to serve.

BEEF AND BROCCOLI STIR-FRY (4 SERVINGS)

1/4 cup soya sauce
½ red or Spanish onion, sliced
1 tbsp garlic, minced
1- ½ pound lean sirloin steak, sliced 1 inch thick
1 tbsp sesame oil
2 tbsp rice vinegar
1 tbsp ginger, minced, 4 cups of broccoli chopped
8 ounces of dried Soba noodles

PER SERVING
466 Calories
11 g Total Fat
46 g Protein
49 g Carbohydrate
99 mg Cholesterol
1,591 mg Sodium

Bring 2 quarts of water to a boil. Meanwhile, heat the ¼ cup of soya sauce in a large pan. Add the onions and garlic, and sauté until opaque. Add beef and sauté, turning often for 7 to 10 minutes. Stir the oil, vinegar, and ginger together, then add to the sauté mixture. Blanche broccoli in the boiling water. Add it to the meat mixture and keep warm. Prepare soba noodles according to package directions. Drain, toss with the beef and broccoli, and serve.

MISO SOUP (8 SERVINGS)

½ tsp sesame oil
1/3 cup shallots or onions, finely chopped
3 tbsp miso paste
1 quart vegetable stock
3 tbsp green onions, sliced for garnish

PER SERVING
107 Calories
3 g Total Fat
4 g Protein
16 g Carbohydrate
1 mg Cholesterol
1,052 mg Sodium

Heat the sesame oil in a pan over medium heat. Add the shallots or onions until translucent. Add the miso and mix well. Add the vegetable stock and bring to a simmer. Reduce heat to low and simmer for 15 minutes. To serve, ladle into bowls and garnish each serving with onions. If desired, add a scoop of non-flavored protein powder just before serving.

LEMON GARLIC CHICKEN (3 SERVINGS)

1/4 cup fresh lemon juice
2 tbsp molasses (Note. buy organic at health food store)
2 tsp Worcestershire sauce
4 garlic cloves, chopped
2 pounds boneless, skinless chicken
1/4 tsp sea salt and black pepper
Lemon wedges and parsley

PER SERVING
153 Calories
4 g Total Fat
21 g Protein
8 g Carbohydrate
86 mg Cholesterol
219 mg Sodium

Combine the first 4 ingredients in a nonreactive bowl and add chicken. Cover and marinate in the refrigerator for 1 hour, turning occasionally. Preheat oven to 425 degrees. Remove chicken from dish, reserving marinade, and arrange in a shallow roasting pan coated with 1-2 tbsp cold pressed olive or safflower oil. Pour reserved marinade over chicken; sprinkle with sea salt and pepper. Bake at 425 degrees for 20 minutes, basting occasionally with marinade. Bake without basting for 20 minutes more or until chicken is done. Serve with lemon wedges and garnish with parsley, if desired.

Basic Vital Health Recipes

CABBAGE SALAD

- ¼ Red Cabbage
- 1 bunch broccoli
- 2-3 medium carrots
- 2 celery sticks
- 2 sheets of Nori seaweed sheets (Note. sold in most Asian food stores)
- ½ ripe Avocado
- 2 slices of Spanish onion

Chop all the raw vegetables first then run them through the food processor. Then dump the shredded vegetable mixture from the processor container into a salad bowl. If you don't have a food processor then you can use a good sharp chopping knife that will cut the cabbage into thin pieces easily. Make sure you have a sharp knife and a good cutting board. Scoop out the ripe inside of the avocado and mix it into the salad. Shred the Nori seaweed sheets into pieces and add in the salad mixture as well. Then add in the various ingredients for the dressing and top with slices of tomatoes and cucumbers for each serving bowl when ready to eat. Cover the salad bowl with plastic or a lid when storing. It can be stored in the fridge for at least 3-4 days.

Dressing

- 2-3 heaping tbsp organic mayonnaise
- 2-3 heaping tbsp Dijon mustard
- 2-3 tsp Tabasco sauce
- 4 tbsp Worcestershire sauce
- 1 tsp black pepper
- 2-3 tbsp garlic powder
- 2 oz balsamic or rice vinegar
- 2 tbsp cold pressed olive oil

TUNA RECIPE

- 2-3 cans tuna (packed in water)
- 1-2 heaping tbsp organic mayonnaise
- 2-3 tbsp of hamburger relish or tomato chutney
- 1 oz diced Spanish onion or green onion
- ½ tsp black pepper
- 1 tbsp garlic powder or 1 clove garlic minced
- 1 tsp dried or fresh parsley
- 1 oz balsamic or rice vinegar
- ½ lemon juice
- ½ tsp paprika or chili powder

Dump the tuna into a glass or ceramic bowl, add all the ingredients and mix well. Then it is ready to eat and goes well on a sandwich or as a side protein dish with salad or eggs. It can also be eaten as a pate on crackers as a snack.

HEALTHY GRAINS

- 2 cups of Quinoa, Brown Rice, Millet, Steel Cut Oats or Pot Barley (Note. sold in most health food, bulk food, Asian food, Middle Eastern or Caribbean food stores)
- 3 cups of water

Usually cook 2 cups of the grains and add 3 cups of water. Bring to a boil and cook at medium heat for about 20 minutes, then simmer at low heat for about 5 minutes or so. You may need to add water as you cook to keep the grains moist. Keep the lid on the pot, partially throughout the cooking times, so the steam can escape and to avoid an over-flow. The grains in North America that are usually eaten as cereals are Oats and Millet. However, I know in some of the African countries Millet is eaten as a main staple like rice with their meat. Brown rice, Quinoa and Pot Barley are consumed here as a staple. However, rice can also be made into a desert like rice pudding or rice flour cakes as some of the Asian recipes do.

KOREAN VEGETABLE SALAD

Choice of Vegetables

- Eggplant
- Cabbage
- Spinach
- Bean Sprouts
- Bok choy
- Water Cress
- Nappa Cabbage

Spices

- 1-2oz Rice Vinegar
- 2-3 Tbsp low sodium Tamari Sauce
- 1-2 Tbsp Sesame Oil

- 2-3 cloves of minced Garlic
- 2-3 sprigs of chopped Green Onion
- 2 Slices of Spanish onion, ½ inch thick/diced
- 1 tsp brown sugar
- 1 tsp sesame seeds (raw or toasted) * toasted for more flavour

Preparation

- Chop vegetables and blanche in boiling water for 2-3 minutes (Note. some vegetables will require more time, some less)
- In a large bowl, mix all spices listed above.
- Combine vegetables and spices.

This Asian marinated salad can be kept fresh in the fridge, cover for up to a week or a week and a half.

LEAN GROUND BEEF, CHICKEN OR TURKEY CASSEROLE

Ingredients

- 3 cloves of garlic, crushed and minced
- 2 pounds of extra lean free range ground beef, chicken or turkey (Note. hormone free)
- 2-3 slices of Spanish onion, cut ½ inch thick, then cut in half
- 1-2 celery diced about ¼ inch
- 1-2 medium sized carrots diced thin
- ½ green or red bell pepper diced
- 3-4 mushrooms cut in chunks
- Add 2 oz medium, Canadian Sherry
- 1-2 oz of rice or balsamic vinegar
- ½ tsp of garlic powder
- ½ tsp of onion powder
- ½ tsp of thyme (fresh if desired)

- ¼ tsp of black pepper
- 1 tsp of brown sugar
- 1 can of tomato sauce

Let it sit for about 15 minutes to allow the meat to marinate in the spices. Then add in the tomato sauce and mix well in a large casserole dish. Put in oven at 350 degree for about 1 hour and a half. Serve with steamed brown rice, potatoes, whole wheat pasta or Sobu (buckwheat) noodles.

LEAN CHICKEN OR FISH BAKE

Ingredients

- 3-4 cloves of garlic, crushed and minced
- 6 pieces of breast chicken, haddock, cod or salmon
- 2-3 slices of Spanish onion, cut ½ inch thick, then cut in half
- 1 medium sized carrot diced thin
- 3 Shitake mushrooms cut in chunks
- Add 2 oz medium, Canadian Sherry
- 1-2 oz of rice or balsamic vinegar
- ½ tsp of garlic powder
- ½ tsp of onion powder
- ¼ tsp of black pepper
- ½ tsp of thyme (fresh if desired)
- 2-3 tsp freshly squeezed lemon
- 2-3 tsp preservative free honey & garlic barbeque sauce
- 1 oz of fresh parsley or cilantro chopped
- 3-4 thin slices of lime or lemon

Let it sit for about 15 minutes to allow the chicken or fish to marinate in the spices and sauce. Preheat oven at 350 degrees for about 20 minutes for the fish or

30-45 minutes for the chicken. Serve with steamed brown rice, potatoes or steamed vegetables.

LINDA'S ALMOND FLOUR GRAVY (4 CUPS)

- 6 Tbsp almond flour
- 4 cups of meat juice
- ¼ tsp sea salt
- ¼ tsp Kirkland organic no salt seasoning
- ¼ granulated garlic

LINDA'S BATTERED WILD SALMON STEAKS

You can buy these wild salmon steaks frozen in a bag at Costco. They usually come with the skin on one side. Beat one egg in a bowl. Put tbsp of olive oil on the pan and heat. Coat the skinless side of the salmon steak with an egg then sprinkle with q tbsp of almond flour. First, put the skin side down on the pan to cook. Once cooked, flip it and peel the cooked skin off with your spatula. Then coat this side with an egg and sprinkle with tbsp of almond flour. Once the other side is cooked, flip this side down to cook. While cooking, sprinkle with sea salt, pepper and Kirkland organic no salt seasoning.

LINDA'S TURNIP

Chop 1 turnip into about 1-2 inch cubes. Put in a deep pot and cook them in boiling water for 20-30 minutes. Once cooked well, drain and put in a large bowl and mash.

- Add 2 tbsp olive oil or 2 tbsp of organic butter
- Add 1 tbsp of maple syrup
- ¼ tsp of sea salt

RAW CRANBERRY SAUCE

- 2 cups of cranberries
- 1 lemon
- 1 orange
- 12 dates
- ¼ cup of maple syrup

Put the two cups of cranberries in the blender or vita mix. Peel the lemon, orange and cut into chunks with the dates. Then pour in the maple syrup, blend until smooth and its ready to serve.

ORGANIC BREAD STUFFING FOR TURKEY

Chop about ¾ of a loaf of organic spelt, kamut, whole wheat or Ezekiel sprouted bread into inch and half pieces and put in a large bowl. This should be enough for a 10-12 pound turkey. Add the rest of the ingredients and mix well, then stuff into the turkey cavity. If there is extra stuffing that you cannot put into the turkey or if you want to make extra stuffing, put it in a glass baking dish. First coat with about tsp of olive oil and bake for about 1 hour at 350 Fahrenheit.

- Add 8-10 prunes chopped in half
- Add 3-4 slices of Spanish onion chopped into about ½ inch chunks
- Add 10-12 olives chopped in half
- Add 1-2 free range egg well beaten
- Add about 1 ½ cups of chicken broth from Non-MSG soup base
- 1 tsp sage (fresh if desired)
- ½ tsp sea salt
- ½ tsp black pepper

LINDA'S BROWN RICE

Measure out 2 cups of brown rice in a measuring cup and put in a strainer. Run water over the rice in the strainer to get the starchy residue off the rice. Then put in a stainless steel pot with 4 cups of water. Mix in about 1 heaping tsp of chicken powdered soup base mix (Non-MSG) in with the water and rice while it is still cold so it does not clump. Chop about 2-3 green onions and mix that into the rice mixture. Set your stove element to high until the rice liquid is boiling then turn down to medium heat for several minutes. Then when you see the rice starting to expand, cook until most of the water is absorbed, turn down the simmer until rice is cooked. Try not to over-cook the rice where it becomes too soft and mushy. Keep it still a little chewy and grainy so that when you re-heat the rice, it is just right. If you would like, sprinkle a tsp of pure sesame oil and ½ tsp of low sodium tamari sauce to taste.

VITAL HEALTH GREEN SMOOTHIE

- Approx. 2 cups of organic spinach
- 2-3 kale leaves (optional)
- ½ a ripe avocado
- 1 organic apple
- 1 pear
- 1-2 inch chunk of fresh ginger

Fill your blender or Vita-mix with about 3 cups of water then add approximately 2 cups of organic spinach chopped. Chop your apples and pears with skin on and core them. Put them in, in addition to the spinach. Chop the ginger into small chunks and add. Cut your avocado in half and peel the hard outer skin off it. You can leave the seed pit in the other half and cover with plastic and keep in fridge. It will last longer with the pit in it. Blend the mixture for a few minutes or just a minute in the Vita-mix until smooth. Then pour yourself a fresh glass where you will get all the nutrients at their optimal level. Pour the rest into a glass container that has a tight cover like a glass mason jar or keep it in the blender glass pitcher with the lid on it in the fridge for later. I find the smoothie usually stays pretty fresh till the next day.

VITAL HEALTH SALAD

First break off the romaine leaves from the core and rinse under cold water. Rinse all the raw vegetables under cold water and pat dry lightly with a tea towel to get most of the water off. If you like, you can add a tbsp of your favourite organic salad dressing to your bowl of salad when you have it.

- Chop the romaine lettuce into two inch chunks into a large bowl with a lid.
- Add one English cucumber chopped in half then into ½ inch pieces
- Add 3-4 celery stalks chopped into ½ inch lengths
- Add one bell pepper chopped
- Add about 12-15 cherry tomatoes
- Add ½ a ripe avocado chopped
- Add about a cup or so of fresh cilantro or parsley chopped
- ½ squeezed fresh lemon
- ¼ tsp of sea salt
- ¼ tsp black pepper
- 2-3 tbsp of cold pressed olive oil

ROASTED ORGANIC CHICKEN

We usually get the frozen organic chicken at Costco. Place the whole chicken in the baking dish first. Put about ½ cup of water with it to make extra gravy if you so desire. Sprinkle all the spices on it; rub the minced pieces of garlic all over the chicken. Then poke holes into the chicken so the spices will absorb into the meat. Then spread the BBQ sauce all over and bake for an hour and half at 350F.

- Add ½ lemon squeezed
- Add 2-3 cloves of fresh garlic minced and spread it over the chicken
- ½ tsp sea salt
- ½ tsp black pepper
- ¼ tsp thyme (fresh if desired)
- 2-3 tbsp of Neal Brother's Organic BBQ Sauce (spread over the whole chicken)

VITAL HEALTH WAKAME SEAWEED SALAD

Put 4 large handfuls of dried seaweed in a large porcelain or glass bowl. Fill bowl with boiled water until all the seaweed is immersed in the water. Let it sit for about 15 minutes or so until the seaweed soaks up the water and expands and comes to its natural state of long stringy seaweed leaves.

Strain well by squeezing the water out of it by hand and put into a mixing bowl.

- Add two to three green onions chopped
- 1-2 garlic clove crushed and minced
- 1 lemon squeezed
- 2-3 tbsp of tamari sauce (low sodium, non-GMO, wheat free soya sauce like taste)
- 1 tsp of raw or roasted sesame seeds
- 2 tbsp of roasted sesame seed oil
- 1 tsp of raw brown sugar (optional)

Mix well and serve with some fish and steamed vegetables or with steamed brown rice and some pickled, fermented vegetables like Kimchi or Dai Kong (pickled Japanese radish)

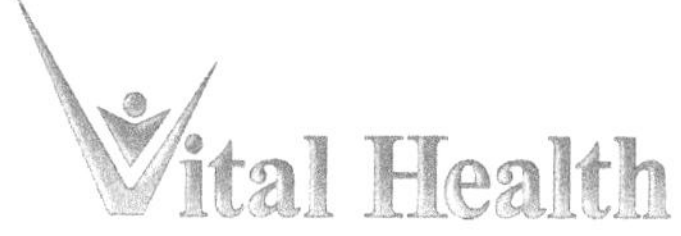

VITAL HEALTH STIR FRY

Dice carrots into slices and fry in a deep dish pan with olive oil and cooking sherry first for a few minutes, then add sliced beef or chicken and cook until half done. Then add in chopped 1 to 1 ½ inch chunks of celery, broccoli, bell pepper, cabbage and water chestnuts. Cook until almost done then add in some chopped in shitake mushrooms. Add a heaping tsp of chicken soup mix (Non-MSG) into cup of boiled water, mix and add to the stir fry mixture. Add in crushed fresh garlic cloves minced with about 2 inch chunk of fresh ginger chopped. Sprinkle in sea salt, black pepper, thyme and some name brand stir fry sauce (preservative free) or some oyster sauce. Mix all ingredients, add water and more of the chicken stock as needed. This recipe gives about 5-6 servings.

- 1-2 carrots sliced 1/4 inch
- 2 celery stalks
- 2 cups broccoli
- 1 bell pepper
- 1 cup cabbage
- 1 cup water chestnuts
- 24 oz beef minute steak, round steak or skinless chicken breasts
- ½ cup shitake mushroom
- 2-3 large fresh garlic cloves
- 2 inch chunk fresh ginger root
- ½ tsp sea salt
- ½ tsp fresh ground pepper
- ¼ thyme (fresh if desired)
- 1-2 heaping tbsp Stir Fry Sauce

ASIAN RICE OR RAMEN NOODLE SOUP

This is a quick light meal that I have modified and made my own version over the years. First you can use either the Thai Kitchen rice noodle package or the organic Ramen noodle packages you can buy at almost any local health food stores. They come with dry rice or organic whole wheat noodles that cook in boiling water in a few minutes and a soup mix package. These packages already have the Asian soup mix ingredients in them. The Thai Kitchen noodle mix is a mixture of sugar, onion powder, garlic, soy protein, spring onions, and spices. The Ramen soup mix is usually a mixture of powdered soybean, miso, shitake mushrooms, onion, garlic, ginger and black pepper. There are also small pieces of wakame seaweed, sea salt and green onion. You first put about 2 ¾ cups of water in a pot and bring to a boil. Add in the soup powder mixture with some chopped green onions, some small pieces of dried Shitake mushrooms and finely diced carrots and let cook for about 2-3 minutes. Then add two of the dry noodle chunks and let cook for another 2 minutes. The rice noodles will cook in about 1-2 minutes and the Ramen wheat noodles will take about 4 minutes. Near the last 2 minutes of the soup cooking with the noodles, add in 1 beaten egg into the soup. Once the noodles are cooked to a chewy consistency take the pot off the heat. Pour the noodles with the liquid into a large deep soup bowl. You can garnish with some thinly sliced raw bell peppers, cucumbers and some Japanese Daikon (pickled radish) on top with the noodles. In addition you can add hot pepper oil that comes with the Thai Kitchen rice noodle package over the noodle soup when you are ready to eat.

I also usually have a side dish of canned salmon and some kimchi (fermented pickled Korean cabbage mixture) with the noodles.

- 2-3 green onions chopped
- 1 inch chunk of carrot sliced thin and diced into very small pieces
- One dried Shitake mushroom broken into ¼ inch pieces
- 1 free range egg beaten in a cup
- Quarter bell pepper sliced into thin strips
- 3-4slices of Daikon (Japanese radish)
- 2 packages of Thai Kitchen Rice Noodle or Organic Ramen Noodle

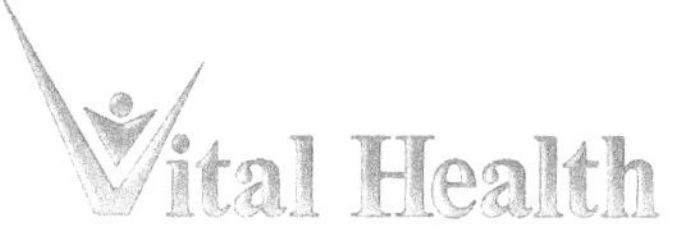

VITAL HEALTH MILLET LOAF

Dry Ingredients

- 1 cup oat or rice flour
- 1/3 cup buckwheat flour
- 1 ½ cup millet flour
- ¼ tsp sea salt
- 2 tsp cinnamon
- ¼ tsp cloves
- ¼ tsp ginger
- 3 ½ tsp baking powder

Wet Ingredients

- 1/3 cup maple syrup
- 1 tbsp vanilla extract
- 1/3 cup butter
- 1/3 cup extra virgin olive oil
- 4 whole eggs
- ¼ cup water
- 1 cup chopped dates

Optional

- 1 cup chopped walnuts or pecans

Preheat oven to 350 F (175 C). Mix all dry ingredients together first. Then add wet ingredients leaving dates and nuts last. Line 9" pan with wax paper then pour in batter. Cook for 45 minutes. It's done when toothpick comes out dry. Remove wax paper and wrap in plastic and foil to keep moist. Allow it to mature for a day.

Supplements

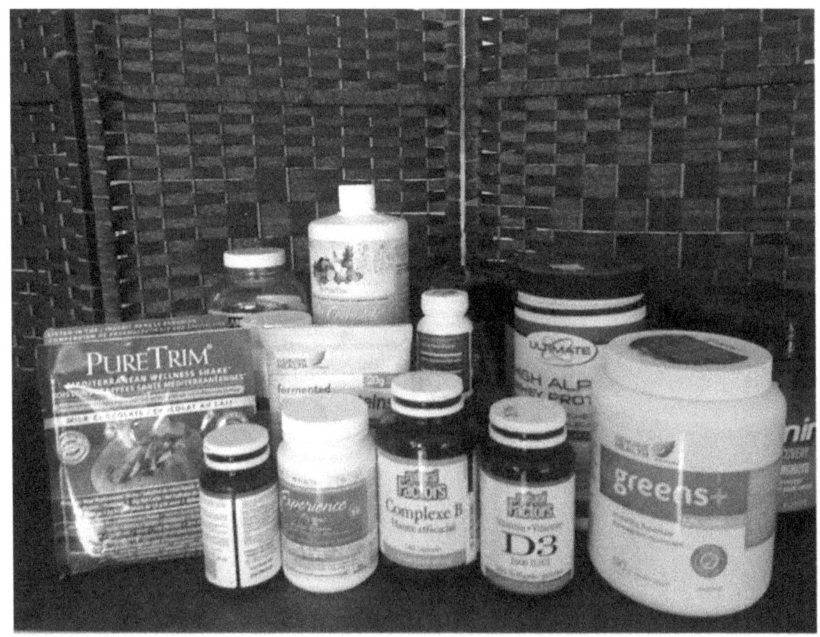

There are an incredible amount of supplements and herbal remedies and formulas out there for us to use and discover. My primary focus of this book is to have you exposed to basic nutrients and supplements that will help you gain a great start in being at your optimal health, keeping your immune system high. I am also trying to provide a realistic but a healthy approach to your eating so you can perform better in the gym, at your work and in your sport. The supplements in this section are the basic ones that

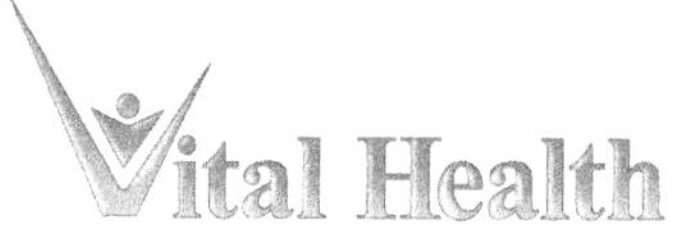

I have used and recommended to clients over the years. I continue to use a select number of them to keep myself nourished and fuelled for my workouts and activity.

VITAMIN B COMPLEX (50 TO 100 MG)

- 1-2 powdered capsules a day with or after breakfast
- The following are the nutrient value and the health benefits of B Vitamins:
- **B1**: Thiamine: function nervous system
- **B2**: Riboflavin: stress
- **B3**: Niacin: brain function, insomnia, digestive
- **B5**: Pantothenic Acid: "anti-stress", effects adrenals
- **B6**: Pyridoxine: hydrochloric acid (HCL), absorption B12, red blood cells (RBC), Metabolize proteins, carbohydrates, selenium, fats, and helps absorb Zinc
- **Folic Acid**: division of cells, utilization of sugar and amino acids, production of nucleic acids, and RBC formation
- **B12**: forms & regenerates RBC, nervous system, growth and development, utilize fats, proteins and carbs, improves memory, concentration and balance, and detoxifies cyanide from foods and tobacco smoke
- Sources of Vitamin Bs: whole grains, beans, oatmeal, eggs, seeds, and green vegetables; usually not enough in food

VITAMIN C (POWDER FORM)

- Water soluble vitamin
- 1-2 tsp per day (approx. 1500 to 3000 mg)
- Take first tsp with 2 oz juice or water with or after breakfast
- Take second tsp with 2 oz water or juice with or after supper
- One of the most important vitamins for the immune system
- Necessary for absorption of Iron, production of stress hormones and helps wounds to heal
- Crucial for growth and repair of blood vessels, cells, gums, bones and teeth

VITAMIN D

- 2000-3000 I.U. of soft gel capsules
- It is a bone builder as it controls and regulates the use of the lime and phosphorus in the body. Rickets are caused from the lack of it.
- It is found in green vegetables, alfalfa and cod liver oil
- It is produced in the body when our skin is exposed to the sun [129]

VITAMIN E

- One 200-400 i.u. capsule a day with or after breakfast
- Oxygen for body, development of nerves and muscles, heals skin, prevents scarring
- Is necessary for fertility and affects both male and female
- Found in wheat, greens peas and olive oil

VITAMIN A (Mega Halibut Liver Oil)

- One 10,000 I.U. capsule of vitamin A per day
- Promotes healthy vision, bones and teeth, maintains strong bones and teeth, and supports body's natural defenses [130]
- Promotes growth, strength, and makes skin and eyes clear
- Children require more of this vitamin than adults; when it's lacking in their diet they cease to grow, keratinisation of the skin, mucous membranes in the respiratory, gastrointestinal and urinary systems can occur [131]
- Eye conditions like night blindness can occur from lack of this vitamin
- This vitamin can be found in spinach, Swiss chard, lettuce, whole milk, butter fat, egg yolk, cabbage, tomatoes, carrots, green peas and sweet potatoes.

CALCIUM & MAGNESIUM

- Approximately 1000 mg in powder form per day for adults up to 50 yrs of age and 1200 mg for adults 51 yrs of age and over
- Builds bones, bone density, muscle, teeth; counteracts acid, aids vitality, soothes nerves
- Liquid Calcium has higher absorption, about 25%

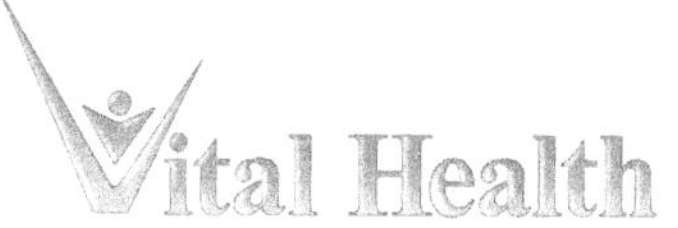

- 1 tbsp per day if meals are high in minerals
- Two 1 tbsp (breakfast and supper) if not eating enough meals with fresh green veg., fruit and protein.
- Calcium is the mineral most likely to be deficient in the average diet. Calcium is the chief supportive element in bones and teeth. Calcium salts make up about 70 percent of bone by weight and give your bone its strength and rigidity. About 99 percent of the calcium in the human body is held in the bones and teeth. The remaining one percent of calcium circulates in the bloodstream, where it performs a variety of important functions. It helps to contract muscles and helps regulate the contractions of the heart. It plays a role in the transmission of nerve impulses and in blood clotting. Calcium is involved in the stimulation of contractions of the uterus during childbirth and in milk production. It also regulates the secretion of various hormones and aids in the functioning of various enzymes within the body. (The Benefits of Calcium, By: Dr. George Obikoya)

POTASSIUM

- One to five 99 mg tablets per day
- Crucial for water balance and protein synthesis, helps form electrolytes, necessary for nerve, muscle function and acts with Sodium to conduct nerve impulses.

SELENIUM (Trace Mineral)

- One 200 mcg capsule a day
- It is an antioxidant and immune system booster, involved in the maintenance of healthy blood cells, healthy skin, healthy eyes, healthy immune system and tissues
- Acts as an antioxidant against free radicals that damage our DNA
- It is often included with Vitamins C and E to help fight against cancer, heart disease and even aging
- It has also been used to fight viral infections and may even slow the progression of AIDS/HIV
- Contributes to good health by promoting normal liver function
- Found in Brazil nuts, poultry, seafood, oats, brown rice and meats

CHROMIUM - (Trace Mineral)

- One 20-35 mcg tablet a day with meals is plenty for adults
- Chromium helps to control blood sugar by increasing its uptake by muscles and organs, controls fat levels and cholesterol levels in the blood
- It is an essential mineral necessary for the formation of Glucose Tolerance Factor, compound that regulates the body's use of glucose and helps to balance blood sugar Chromium is also used in the metabolism and storage of fats, proteins, and carbohydrates by the body
- I would only recommend to take an extra Chromium supplement if you are deficient
- Deficiency symptoms: cold sweats, dizziness, irritability when hungry, cold hands, need for sleep, drowsy during the day, addiction to sweet foods, frequent urination and excessive thirst
- Food sources: Brewer's yeast, whole wheat bread, vegetables like broccoli, potatoes, and green beans, fruits, beef, poultry, rye bread, oysters, peas, shredded wheat breakfast cereal, and wheat germ [132]

MULTI ENZYME FULL SPECTRUM

- One 525 mg capsule with each meal is helpful or as directed by physician
- Periodically , I use enzyme supplements made by Natural Factors to help in digestion when I am consuming a lot of meals in one day with high amounts of meat and complex carbohydrates. It is made from plant based enzymes. It helps your digestive system work easier at breaking down all the foods you are consuming. This is really helpful if you are not getting enough raw vegetables in your diet. It helps aid with protein, carbohydrate, dairy and fat digestion.

For carbohydrate digestion it contains:

Amylase enzyme
Cellulase enzyme
Lactase enzyme
Maltase enzyme

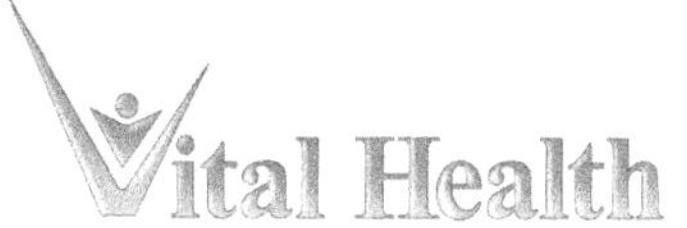

Sucrase
Hemicellulase

For Protein Digestion:
Protease I
Protease II
Protease III
Peptizyme SPTM
Bromelain
Papain

For Lipid Digestion:
Lipase [133]

COENZYME Q10

- 30-200 mg soft gel per day is sufficient
- Higher doses may be taken for specific conditions
- It is a fat soluble antioxidant so it is absorbed more effectively when taken with meals containing fat. This compound occurs naturally in your body, but as you get older and acquire nutritional deficiencies, or get sick, your body produces less and less of this essential anti-oxidant. Studies have shown, that with a Coenzyme Q10 deficiency of approximately 25%, you start to experience serious metabolic health problems. And at a 75% Coenzyme Q10 deficiency – death is almost certain! Coenzyme Q10 plays a key role in the production of adenosine triphosphate (ATP) which is needed for cellular energy production. Coenzyme Q10 is also a super antioxidant that helps guard you against damage from free radicals.
- Main benefits are: stimulates your body's metabolism for weight loss, suppresses gingival inflammation, improves sperm mobility and protects against free radicals, improves symptoms in cardiac and congestive heart failure patients and significantly enhances immune function. In various other studies,

Coenzyme Q10 provided tremendous benefits in lowering high blood pressure and helped with angina, and congestive heart failure.[134]

PROBIOTICS

- One capsule of over 1 billion lactobacillus and other good bacteria is the recommended dose. Best time to take it is in the morning with your breakfast or an extra one with meals if your digestion is weak.
- Many of the probiotic supplements lose over 90% of their potency in the first 30 days because they don't make it past the stomach in the body. However, I recommend you try a probiotic I use called Synergy by PureTrim where the good bacteria is in a special capsule that does not breakdown until it reaches the digestive tract so you get more addition of the good bacteria into your system. Also, they have added extra plant enzymes and an antioxidant herbal blend with it to maximize your digestion even more. Again their website if you want to order is: vitalcleanse.puretrim.com.
- An estimated 100 trillion microorganisms representing more than 500 different species inhabit every normal, healthy bowel. These microorganisms are very helpful. These gut-dwelling bacteria keep pathogens (harmful microorganisms) in check, aid digestion and nutrient absorption, and contribute to immune function. Probiotics can help gastrointestinal ailments, vaginal and urinary infections in women, crohns, and irritable bowel syndrome (IBS).

OMEGA-3 (liquid or soft gel capsules)

- 2 tbsp or 3 soft gel capsules per day with breakfast for average adult
- I recommend 3 soft gel capsules or 1 tbsp with or after breakfast and 3 soft gel capsules or 1 tbsp with supper if you have joint issues or doing intense training in the gym, practicing in a professional sport like football, hockey, long distance running, cycling or tri-athlete training where the joints are being used excessively and your energy output is very high.
- Our body cannot produce omega-3's so we need to get it from food sources. It is a natural anti-inflammatory, treats arthritis, asthma and various skin conditions like dry skin, psoriasis, dry eyes and excessive thirst. Omega-3 thins the

blood to prevent clotting, and helps prevent cardiovascular disease. It has anti-inflammatory and anti-coagulant properties as well as many other important health benefits. They are involved in the formation of cellular membranes, development of brain activity, and the manufacturing of substances necessary for blood pressure regulation, blood vessel elasticity, and inflammation and immune responses of the body.

- Omega-6 is also essential and is transformed into leukotrienes, pro-inflammatory molecules that promote coagulation and cell growth. They defend against pathogens and also repair lesions and cell tearing from wounds. However, we get more than enough omega-6's since it is present in vegetable oils, and as you may already know much of our foods have vegetable oil in them. They are in salad dressings, our breads, crackers, baked goods, restaurant vegetables, soups, etc. Therefore most people consume over ten times more omega-6 than omega-3. We get a lot of omega-3 from Mackerel, Salmon, Sardines and Herring. However, if you do not eat fresh fish regularly, about 2-3 times a week, then I suggest you take an omega-3 supplement daily as prescribed in this section.

CHLOROPHYLL

- 1 to 2 tsp with 1- 2 cups of water
- Chlorophyll is the green pigment found in all plants and algae. It absorbs sunlight and uses its energy to synthesize carbohydrate CO2 and water. It is the life blood of the plant. It is a good source of iron, decreases mucus, detoxifies the liver and accelerates re-growth of cells. It Inhibits cancer causing elements, purifies, detoxifies the liver,
- cleanses the body, and eliminates toxic pollutants and even heavy metals.
- It can be used as an antiseptic for the intestinal tract, rebuilds damaged bowel tissue,
- eliminates mucous, removes harmful bacteria, and reduces acidity.
- Chlorophyll helps to rebuild and replenish our red blood cells, boosting our energy and increasing our well-being. Also, it has the power to regenerate our bodies at the molecular and cellular level and is known to help cleanse the

body, fight infection, help heal wounds, promote the health of the circulatory, digestive, immune, and detoxification systems.

- The consumption of this amazing substance increases the number of red blood cells and, therefore, increases oxygen utilization by the body. It reduces binding of carcinogens to DNA in the liver and other organs and breaks down calcium oxalate stones for elimination, which are created by the body for the purpose of neutralizing and disposing excess acid. It also decreases mucus, detoxifies liver and inhibits abnormal growth in liver and colon cells. [135]

GREENS PLUS

- Two heaping tsp with ounce of water, juice or fresh veg. / fruit juice from juice machine
- This is a very potent concentrated green powder made from plants, algae, vegetables, fruits, wheat grass, bee pollen, and caretenoids. It is a multi-mineral in plant and vegetable food base form. It helps support the immune system, increase energy naturally, enhance mental acuity, cleanse and detoxify the body and provides an alkaline pH state. I personally take it as a supplement to make up for the five servings of green vegetables that many of us do not get consistently on a daily basis. It comes in powder or capsule form and in different fruit flavours for those who cannot handle just the greens taste.
- It is a blend of 29 different Superfoods. This mixture contains three types of algae, valuable antioxidants and a blend of vitamins and minerals. It does not contain any fillers, preservatives, fat or sugar. Greens Plus contains substantial vitamin and mineral properties. One such ingredient is Bee Pollen. This ingredient is known for being rich in antioxidants. There is the possibility of an allergic reaction to the Royal Jelly and bee pollen if someone is allergic to bees. Furthermore, it contains an abundance of Vitamin K which can be problematic for people that take blood thinners. It also contains licorice root which may elevate blood pressure. 136
- For a comprehensive list of ingredients, please visit www.greensplus.com.

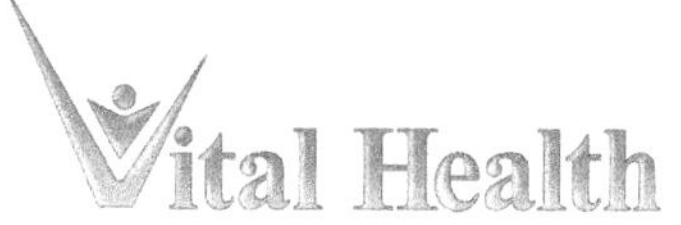

CHLORELLA (Single-celled fresh-water green algae)

- 1-2 capsules per day or ½ tsp per day with an oz of water or veg/fruit juice
- Detoxifies, cleanses the body of harmful toxins such as pesticides and heavy metals.
- Protects body cells from free radical damage, increase immune system.
- Provides vitamins, minerals, amino acids and nutritional elements for the body

JOINT CARE – 1000 mg capsules

- One capsule 2- 3 times per day before, after or in between each meal
- It contains glucosamine which stimulates production of collagen, chondriotin sulfate which prevents cartilage breakdown and Methyl-Sulfonyl-Methane (MSM) that increases cell, tissue permeability which reduces joint pain.

DAILY COMPLETE (liquid vitamin from Pure Trim)

- 1 capful with 2 oz. water or other juices with breakfast once per day
- Contains 194 vitamins, mineral, organic fruits, vegetables, antioxidants, enzymes, amino acids and Mediterranean herbs
- Contains Phytoplankton Blend that contains hundreds of potent phytochemicals, organic anti-aging Mediterranean super seed mixture and is 60% absorption
- Secondary alternative to juicing with juicer (Available at: vitalcleanse.puretrim.com)

ECHINACEA TINCTURE (Vogel)

- 10 drops in 2 oz of water or juice 3 times per day, or 10 drops under the tongue
- Anti-viral, anti-bacterial for prevention of colds, congestion
- Do not use more than 8 weeks at a time because immune suppression may occur. [137]

PURE GARDENS SKIN CREAM (Pure Trim)

- Helps smooth out facial lines, age spots, skin texture and moisturizes skin
- Contains antioxidants, softens dry, rough spots

- No added chemicals
- Helps heal infections, cuts and wounds
- (Listed in the Canadian Compendium of Pharmaceuticals and Specialties, CPS)
- Available at: vitalcleanse.puretrim.com

NATURAL SKIN CARE OIL (Aura Cacia, Bioforce, or Now)

- 4 to 6 drops for your face and body after a bath or shower, before you towel dry your skin.
- From Grape Seed, Apricot Seed, Jojoba, etc.
- Contains Vitamin E, tones and protects, nourishes skin with fatty acids, anti-oxidants and vitamins

PURE SWEET ALMOND OIL

- Just a size of a quarter in your hand is enough for your face. You can apply to other dry areas of your body after a shower while your pores are still open.
- You can buy this oil at Middle Eastern food stores or at your local health food store. It is a good moisturizer for face or body. Keep in a glass bottle as much as possible.

TEA TREE OIL

- This is a good herbal antiseptic that everyone should have in their bathroom. You can put a few drops on your footh; rub it in around your toes if you struggle with athlete's foot. It helps prevent the spreading of bacterial conditions on the skin. Also, it works well for tooth aces and tooth infections, where you can rub in a few drops right on the tooth and gums. It actually relieves the pain.

STRONG IODINE SOLUTION

- Since we in the west do not get enough iodine in our foods, I recommend taking some every day. The best way to absorb iodine is to put an open bottle upside down tightly placed against your lower forearm, near your wrist and then position the bottle right side up again. This will leave a dark brown iodine spot on your skin. Then rub both of your forearms together and it will absorb quickly. The brand I use is by a company called Laboratories Atlas Inc. You should also be able to get it at your local pharmacy.

BEESWAX FACIAL CREAM

- This is a cream I have started to use for different areas of my body that has a tendency to show up in the winter as eczema patches. It's made from 100% natural bee's wax and grape seed oil. It can be used for rough dry hands. It is also good for eczema and psoriasis. You can notice a difference within days. Many people with skin conditions are now symptom free using this amazing cream! [138]
- It is made locally here near Ottawa by a company called Bee Sweet. These products are available at: beesweetontario.com

SOLID PERFUMES

- I have stopped using colognes which have chemicals and alcohol in them. I use this wonderful solid perfume mixture called Ganesha's Garden Solid Perfume. Many of the health stores carry them. Their website is: betweenheavenandearth.ca.

HARMONY (Pure Trim)

- 2 tsp with 4-6 oz warm water, as a tea
- Improves overall well-being, body balancing ingredients, helps with Acid Indigestion
- Liquid Mediterranean herbal formula over 285 yrs old
- (Listed in the Canadian Compendium of Pharmaceuticals and Specialties, CPS)
- Available at: 6vitals.puretrim

FEMALE BALANCE (Pure Trim)

- Mediterranean herbal formula
- For women experiencing menstrual symptoms take one capsule in the morning or evening for the first two days. Then gradually increase to 1-2 capsules two times a day in the morning and evening.
- For women experiencing menopausal symptoms take one capsule in the morning or evening for the first few days. Then gradually increase to 1-2 capsules two times a day in the morning and evening.
- Helps females with the unique mild symptoms of PMS and Menopause
- (Listed in the Canadian Compendium of Pharmaceuticals and Specialties, CPS)
- Available at: 6vitals.puretrim

VITAL HEALTH COLD REMEDY

- 1-2 oz water
- 1 tsp or squirt of Liquid Chlorophyll
- 10 drops of Echinacea and Golden Seal
- 10 drops of oil of Oregano
- 1 tsp of Powdered Vitamin C
- Stir well and take every 2-3 hours until you feel the cold or flu symptoms diminish

Strength, Recovery and Building Supplements

CREATINE MONOHYDRATE (powder)

- Two 5 g scoops of creatine on training days, approx. 1 hour before training, and 1 hour after workout
- One 5 g on day-off of training in the morning with breakfast or after meals
- Increases muscular strength, lean muscle mass, and gives faster recovery during exercise

GLUTAMINE

I recommend 5-10 g of Glutamine with 2 oz of water or juice at bedtime every day or 3 times a day depending on your level of training. Glutamine produces better body recuperation and strengthens the immune system. It increases muscular volume, decreases catabolism and regulates protein synthesis, and degradation. Glutamine is best known for being an "anti-catabolic" agent. What this means is that rather than directly promoting the growth of new muscle tissue, glutamine works by preserving the muscle tissue that you have already built. You see, muscle breakdown is occurring all the time. This naturally happens when you train intensely, when you don't provide your body with enough protein or during your sleep. This process is completely natural and is to be expected. However, if you are training and eating properly, then your body is also synthesizing new muscle tissue throughout the day. Your overall muscle gains can be calculated by taking the rate of muscle growth and subtracting the rate of muscle breakdown. Glutamine helps by minimizing the rate of muscle breakdown, resulting in greater overall net gains in muscle mass. It also has a very positive effect on the immune system. Not only are your muscles heavily stressed from your workouts, but your entire immune system is stressed as well. Glutamine will help you to recover quicker in between your workouts and will also help to prevent you from getting sick. (The-Dramatic-Muscle-Building-Benefits-Of-Glutamine by Sean Nalewanyj)

WHEY ISOLATE

Whey isolate is a protein extracted from the whey of the milk, where there hardly is any lacto or dairy characteristics left in the whey isolate. Therefore, fewer calories, less fat, but high in protein. It is a high quality protein that allows quick assimilation and positive nitrogenic retention which helps muscles grow faster. It's low in fat and lactose.

- 2 scoops in one blender with 2 ½ - 3 cups of water, 1 banana and add 4-6 oz of frozen or fresh strawberries, blueberries or fruit of your choice
- You will need 2 to 3 blender shakes per day for people on intense training schedules, trying to gain more lean muscle mass, and who need more calories.

WHEY CONCENTRATE

This is concentrated powder of the whey of the milk. Whey protein began its popularity with athletes and body builders, but has continued to grow in popularity as an aid for many health concerns. Whey protein definitely helps to increase lean muscle mass. Without protein, you may spend hours in the gym and never increase your lean muscle mass simply because you cannot grow a muscle without protein. It is useful for weight loss, specifically fat loss. Whey protein is the most easily absorbed, easy to utilize protein, with the most protein per serving.

- 2 scoops in one blender with 2 ½ - 3 cups of water, 1 banana and add 4-6 oz of frozen or fresh strawberries, blueberries or fruit of your choice
- You will need 2 to 3 blender shakes per day for people on intense training schedules, trying to gain more lean muscle mass, and who need more calories.

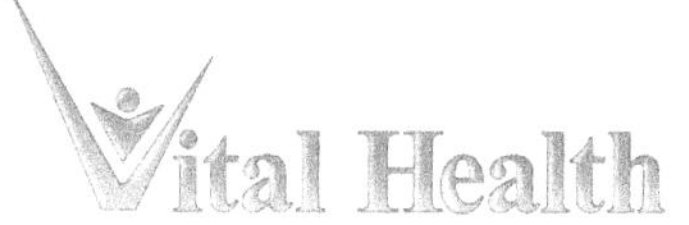

INDOL-3-CARBINOL (I3C):

Helps to preserve testosterone from converting to estrogen; extract from cruciferous vegetables. Take 200 mg twice a day.

TRIBULUS TERRESTRIS

Increases luteinizing hormone (LH) and dehydroepiandrosterone (DHEA) which boosts testosterone. Take 500 to 1,000 mg per day, in between meals.

TONGKAT ALI (Eurycoma Longifolia or LongJack)

Known as the "Asian Viagra"; raises testosterone and helps with weight-loss. Make sure it is a standardized extract of 50:1. Take 200 mg per day.

ARGININE

Improves testosterone levels. Take 3,000 mg per day between meals at bedtime.

ZINC

Maintains testosterone levels in the blood. Also it increases LH hormone activity which stimulates the production of testosterone. Zinc also inhibits testosterone conversion to estrogen. Take 25 to 50 mg per day.

MACA POWDER

Boosts energy, libido and strength. Take 1 heaping tsp and mix in your protein shake once a day, in the morning at the beginning of your day.

PURE TRIM (Vegetarian Meal Replacement)

- Box of 10 packs

This is a low carbohydrate, high protein blend from vegetable pea and brown rice that is a hormonally balanced meal replacement. It's made up of pea and brown rice, contains super greens, essential fatty acids, anti-stress blend and plant calcium to help boost overall weight loss and wellness. These are rich delicious shakes that are low carbohydrate, high protein, 225 calories per blender of shake, less than 1 gram of sugar sweetened with stevia and leaves you full for hours. You just add water, so it's easy to make. It's available at: vitalcleanse.puretrim.com

Recipe: Mix 1 pack with 3 cups of water, 2 ice cubes, 4-6 oz of low sugar fruits like strawberries, blueberries, etc.

One pack makes about three 8 oz cups. Have a 12 oz glass of the shake instead of breakfast or dinner or both. If you want to experience weight-loss then just replace your breakfast or supper with a large shake. Still have a good lunch of meat and vegetables. Refer to the weight loss section of the book for more details.

BRANCH CHAIN AMINO ACIDS (BCAA)

- 3 scoops with 2 oz juice 1-3 times a day between meals.

This is a highly concentrated amino acid blend for those on severe weight-loss or weight gain program. It's very low in fat and calories. The main use is for the purpose of maintaining muscle or increasing muscle.

T&T (Organika)

- Natural Libido Product for Men
- Made from Tribulus Terrestris (Puncture Vine), standardized 40% Saponins
- Enhances Testosterone production naturally
- Improves erectile function by increasing the male hormone Testosterone naturally

Healthy Treats List Explained

I have provided on the next page in the Appendices a list of fairly healthy treats or meals you can have when you are outside, traveling or running around doing your errands in your city or town. If you live in a very remote area then you may have to drive to the nearest commercialized town or city to buy these treats and meals. I sometimes personally eat these foods when I am too busy to cook. There still is good nutritional value in the foods so this is why I provided this for you to use.

Appendix I

HEALTHY TREATS LIST

- 1 Chicken Shawarma pita sandwich with 1 tsp of garlic sauce
- 1 organic almond & honey croissant made from whole grain flour (Note. usually at organic bakeries)
- 1-2 oz of fresh hummus made with healthy oils and pure ingredients
- 1 small decaffeinated skim milk or almond milk Latte with 1 tsp of raw sugar and 1 tsp of soya or organic milk
- 1 medium bowl of Vietnamese rice noodle soup with chicken or sea food
- 1 order of Vietnamese rice shrimp or beef wraps with 1 tsp of peanut sauce
- 1 baked chicken & vegetable Samosa
- 1-2 baked tofu cutlets, vegetable burgers or tofu burgers with 1 tsp of relish or tomato chutney
- 4 oz of plain low fat organic yogurt with 4 oz low sugared fruit like kiwis, melons, strawberries, blueberries, apples, nectarines, peaches or papaya
- 1-2 whole wheat Chapati or Roti wrap with 2-4 oz nitrate-free smoked turkey, ham or home-made roast beef, sliced tomato, cucumbers, 1 tsp of low fat mayonnaise, ½ tsp of Dijon mustard and 1 tsp of tomato chutney or relish
- 8 oz of roasted chicken with 1 tsp of tomato chutney or relish and 4oz of deli sweet potato salad with raisins and 4oz of deluxe deli bean salad

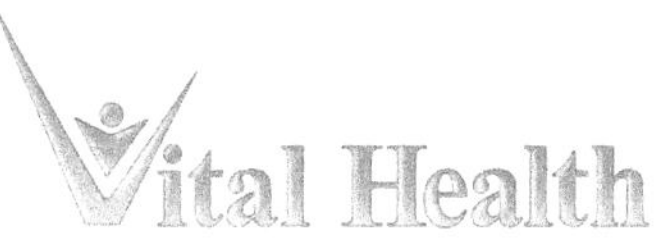

- Serving of 12 oz of organic squash or tomato soup with ½ tsp of cinnamon sprinkled on top and 1-2 slice of Chapati or 2-4 whole grain crackers
- A serving of ½ of a Lebanese chicken plate dinner with 1 tsp of garlic sauce or sweet sauce and 1-2 oz of hummus
- 2 oz of sliced low fat Allegro cheese melted on one slice of brown rice flour bread toasted, with a slice of tomato, cucumber and Spanish onion on it
- 2-4 whole grain crackers with ½ tsp of organic almond butter and ½ tsp of Crofter's organic jam sweetened with grape juice
- 8-12 Tortilla chips with 2-4 oz of Black Bean and Corn Salsa (PC at Loblaws)
- Prepared fresh sushi meal box or a fresh sushi meal at a local Japanese Restaurant

Appendix II

HEALTH TIPS

I felt this section would be useful to know since it shows the effects of the main elements, minerals, vitamins, acids, and antioxidants in our foods. How they work and what happens when we are deficient in them. Also it's good to know what food sources contain that particular element, vitamin, mineral and antioxidant that your body needs.

SULPHUR

- **Food containing:** Brussels sprouts, cabbage, endive, mustard greens, leeks, onions, lobsters, beef, raspberries, loganberries, rhubarb, spinach, watercress, carrots, and radishes.
- **Effects:** acts on the liver, acts on the blood vessels and nerve tissue, beautifies complexion, regulates innervations, helps the hair, nails, skin, cornea of eye, purifies and tones the system, and warms the skin.
- **Deficiency in:** causes weakness and pains everywhere, weak vocal cords, strained nerves, volcanic emotions, flow of blood to the brain, skin eruption, and puffiness under the skin.

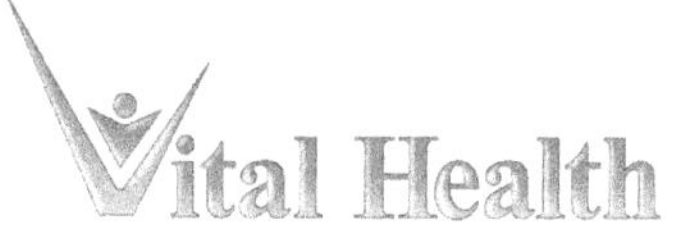

PHOSPHORUS

- **Foods containing:** raw egg yolk, whole barley, whole wheat, corn, lamb, nuts, lobsters, mushrooms, mustard greens, raisins, pumpkin, whole rice, rye meal, milk, and squash.
- **Effects:** acts on the bone and brain; strengthens mental powers; improves nutrition of nerve tissue, especially heart tissue; agent of life and growth; and aids in growth of hair.
- **Deficiency in:** causes neuralgia, wakefulness at night, numbness of the skin, poor hair growth, shallow breathing, dislike of exertion, and melancholy.

POTASSIUM

- **Foods containing:** dried apples, apple peel, dandelion, watercress, lima beans, red beets, parsley, cabbage, potato skin, broccoli, cabbage, figs, peaches, coconut, celery, cucumbers, eggplant, beaten egg white, greens peppers, parsnip, raisins, rhubarb, spinach, romaine lettuce, Swiss chard, watermelons, and whole wheat.
- **Effects:** digests fats, produces alkalinity, stimulates liver, and controls the muscular system.
- **Deficiency in:** causes nervousness, periodic headaches, chills and thirst, valvular ailments, gnawing in stomach, muscular anemia, and muscular fatigue.

CALCIUM

- **Foods containing:** milk, cheese, shrimp, apricots, figs, cabbage, celery, cauliflower, spinach, beets, bran, raw egg yolk, lemons, onions, cranberries, radishes, cottage cheese, Swiss chard, dates, string beans, endives, and cucumbers.
- **Effects:** builds bone, muscle, teeth, etc., counteracts acid, aids vitality, soothes the nerves and decreases nervousness, and stimulates courage.
- **Deficiency in:** causes lack of will power, inward fears, poor teeth, nervousness, pasty complexion, and tired feeling with little exertion.

SODIUM

- **Foods containing:** apples, celery, asparagus, string beans, turnips, carrots, beets, cabbage, egg whites, oysters, crabs, lobsters, strawberries, Swiss chard, oatmeal, coconut, and figs.
- **Effects:** checks fermentation, prevents clotting of blood; stimulates the spleen, regulates heat in body fluids; excites bowels and stomach to greater action; and neutralizes acids.
- **Deficiency in:** causes delayed digestion, frontal headaches, dry skin, sleepiness during the day and wakefulness at night, joints crack, and acid conditions.

MAGNESIUM

- **Foods containing:** mustard greens, grapefruit, oranges, figs, sugar beets, whole wheat, corn, goat milk, wild rice, plums, dandelion greens, and coconuts.
- **Effects:** promotes cell building in nerve matter; promotes excretions; aids constipation; steadies the nerves, and overcomes brain fog, cools the liver and reduces temper.
- **Deficiency in:** causes poor digestion, constipation, sleeplessness, torpid liver, and fits of temper.

SILICON

- **Foods containing:** asparagus, cucumbers, spinach, lettuce, dandelion greens, onions, whole rice, parsnips, tomatoes, barley, oats, figs, and strawberries.
- **Effects:** protective to skin and body; increases hair growth; regulates enamel on teeth, powerful antiseptic; stimulates brain; gives grace to body, sparkle to eyes, and beauty promoter.
- **Deficiency in:** causes poor hair growth, nail ailments, sleeplessness, varicose veins, morbid imagination, nervous dyspepsia, low body temperature, mental strain, soreness in thighs, heat pressure, skin blotches, and low healing power.

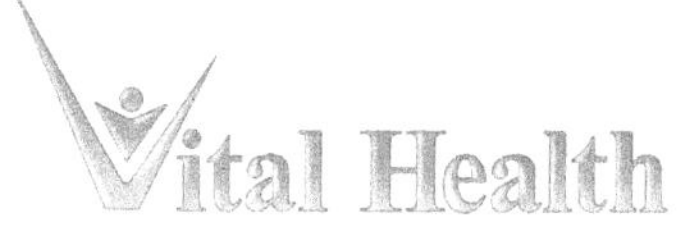

CHLORINE

- **Foods containing:** Raw meat juice, cow or goat milk, kale, beets, radishes, spinach, rye flour, coconut, tomatoes, and ripe olives.
- **Effects:** expels wastes, lowers fat, sugar and starch metabolism, cleans and purifies the system.
- **Deficiency in:** causes scanty hair growth, clumsy movements of muscles, soft teeth, obesity, yellowish skin, and coated tongue.

FLUORINE

- **Foods containing:** goat milk, egg yolk, endives, cabbage, cauliflower, Brussell sprouts, avocado, tomatoes, watercress, raw sea food, and cheese.
- **Effects:** active in bone strength; sets strongly on spleen, teeth, enamel of teeth; protects us from germs and infections; preserves youthfulness in youth and old age, and is bone and teeth insurance.
- **Deficiency in:** causes difficulty in thinking, heavy morning sleep, strong appetite, poor teeth, disorderly mind and habits; and pus and toxins are in the brain, bone and blood.

MANGANESE

- **Foods containing:** watercress, acorns, chestnuts, almonds, rye flour, almost all nuts, oatmeal, raw egg yolks, parsley, and nasturtium leaves.
- **Effects:** acts upon the nerve and brain cells; increases the ability to read small print and to notice objects at a greater distance; strengthens memory; and quickens coordination of thought and action.
- **Deficiency in:** causes profuse perspiration, eye conditions, poor memory, rushing sounds in the head, tension in abdomen, tendency for breast conditions, and nervousness.

NITROGEN-HYDROGEN-CARBON

- **Foods containing:** all sea foods, milk, cheese, beans, lean meats, eggs, and lentils.
- **Effects:** proteins build body and tissue.
- **Deficiency in:** causes lack in tissue replacement and warmth.

VITAMIN F

- Prevents stunted growth, loss of appetite, nervousness, and paralysis
- Is found in lettuce, green vegetables, etc.

DIGESTIVE ENZYMES

Nearly 75 percent of the body's immune defenses are located in the digestive tract, making optimum digestive function the key to overall health. In order to ensure proper digestion, your body requires a dependable supply of digestive enzymes. The chemicals released into the digestive tract can break down food by breaking apart the bonds that hold nutrients together. The body progressively loses its ability to produce enzymes with major drops occurring roughly every ten years of life. Enzymes are energized protein molecules essential for the digestion of food, brain stimulation, tissue, cell and organ repairing and generating cellular energy.

- **Food Sources:** fresh vegetables and fruits, especially the leafy dark green and yellow, orange vegetables like sweet yellow, and orange peppers.
- **Symptoms of low enzymes in the digestive tract:** Heartburn, gas, constipation, bloating, allergies, ulcers, and lack of energy.

ALPHA LIPOIC ACID

Alpha-lipoic acid (ALA), also known as lipoic acid (or thioctic acid), is a sulfur-containing fatty acid found inside every cell of the human body. The main function of alpha-lipoic acid is to generate the energy required to keep living organisms alive and functioning. Lipoic acid plays a key role in a variety of vital energy-producing reactions in the body that turn glucose (blood sugar) into energy.

Alpha-lipoic acid is a potent biological antioxidant that has been shown to slow the oxidative damage in cells, and in many cases stabilize or even reverse cell damage. Alpha-lipoic acid is so effective as an anti-oxidant because it works on both water and fat-soluble free radicals that cause oxidation and cell damage in the body. Helps combat aging, neutralizes free radicals, and helps regenerate vitamin C, E to increase their effectiveness to scavenge free radicals (Kagan V, Khan S, Swanson C, et al. Antioxidant action of thioctic acid and dihydrolipoic acid. Free Radical Bio. Med 1990;9S:15)

GLUTATHIONE

"Glutathione is a very interesting, very small molecule that's [produced by the body and] found in every cell," says Gustavo Bounous, MD, director of research and development at Immunotec and a retired professor of surgery at McGill University in Montreal, Canada. "It's the body's most important antioxidant because it's within the cell." Because glutathione exists within the cells, it is in a prime position to neutralize free radicals. The strong antioxidant effect of glutathione helps keep cells running smoothly. Doctor Bounous and another glutathione expert, Jeremy Appleton, ND, say it also helps the liver remove chemicals that are foreign to the body, such as drugs and pollutants.

"These statements have not been evaluated by the Food and Drug Administration. These programs and products are not intended to diagnose, treat, cure or prevent any disease. This manual should be used with the guidance of a health professional to get the best results."

Appendix III

HIGH NUTRIENT FOODS

CRUCIFEROUS VEGETABLES

- Contains phytonutrient isothiocyanates which fight tumors, breast, prostate and colon cancer. [139]
- Broccoli, cauliflower, Brussell sprouts, kale, cabbage, radish, turnip and watercress

FLAX SEEDS

- Has lignans a phytoestrogen compound which scavenges free radicals in the body and has antiagiogenic properties which stop tumors from forming new blood vessels

GREEN TEA

- Filled with polyphenols like flavonoids and catechins which function as powerful antioxidants that reduce formation of free radicals in the body, protecting cells and molecules from damage. [140]

OLIVE OIL

- Has polyphenols that have anti-inflammatory, anti-cancer and anti-coagulant properties and also help in controlling insulin levels [141]

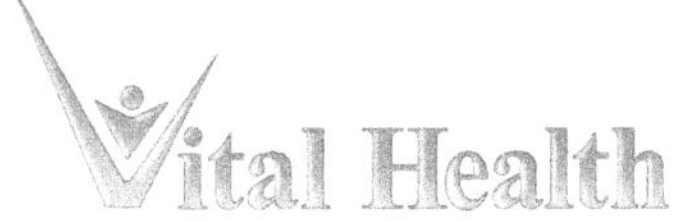

AVOCADO

- High source of potassium, rich in vitamin K, B, C, and E; mostly monounsaturated fat which is good fat [142]

ORGANIC APPLE

- Contains strong antioxidant, quercetin, flavonoids, reduces osteoporosis, heart disease, cancer, stroke, and type 2 diabetes

SALBA GRAIN

- This is a gluten free ancient grain, high source of omega-3, high fibre, minerals, magnesium, potassium, folic acid, iron, and calcium; has all the amino acids [143]

ALMONDS

- Has flavonoids that work with vitamin E to protect artery walls from damage, contains phosphorous which helps strong bones and teeth; lowers the rise in blood sugar and insulin after meals; alkalize the body; contains riboflavin and L-carnitine that boosts brain activity. [144]

CINNAMON

- Lowers blood sugar levels in type 1 and 2 diabetes, has insulin balancing effect

OAT BRAN

- Has vitamin E, zinc, selenium, iron, manganese, magnesium; high in protein, fibre, balances sugar, and insulin levels.

BUCKWHEAT

- This is a gluten free grain, alkaline food, good for celiac, gluten sensitive diets, and people with food allergies; and it can be used as an alternative to rice or served as a cereal

ORGANIC PLAIN YOGURT

- This is a natural source of probiotic, promotes healthy bacterial balance; metabolism of estrogen [145]

POMEGRANATE

- Has anti-cancer, anti-inflammatory and antioxidant properties

TURMERIC

- Naturally decreases inflammatory pain and swelling

GINGER

- Helps with nausea, anti-inflammatory and help with blood flow

DARK CHOCOLATE

- Boosts our endorphins, feelings of attraction, excitement and love; triggers anandamide which gives a feeling of a natural high.

Appendix IV

FIT FOR LIFE

Food Combining Chart For Complete and Efficient Digestion
(Harvey & Marilyn Diamond's Fit For Life)

Foods Properly Combined streamline digestion, promote weight loss and energize and strengthen your entire body. Proteins and Starches eaten together tend to spoil in the stomach leading to indigestion, weight gain and fatigue.

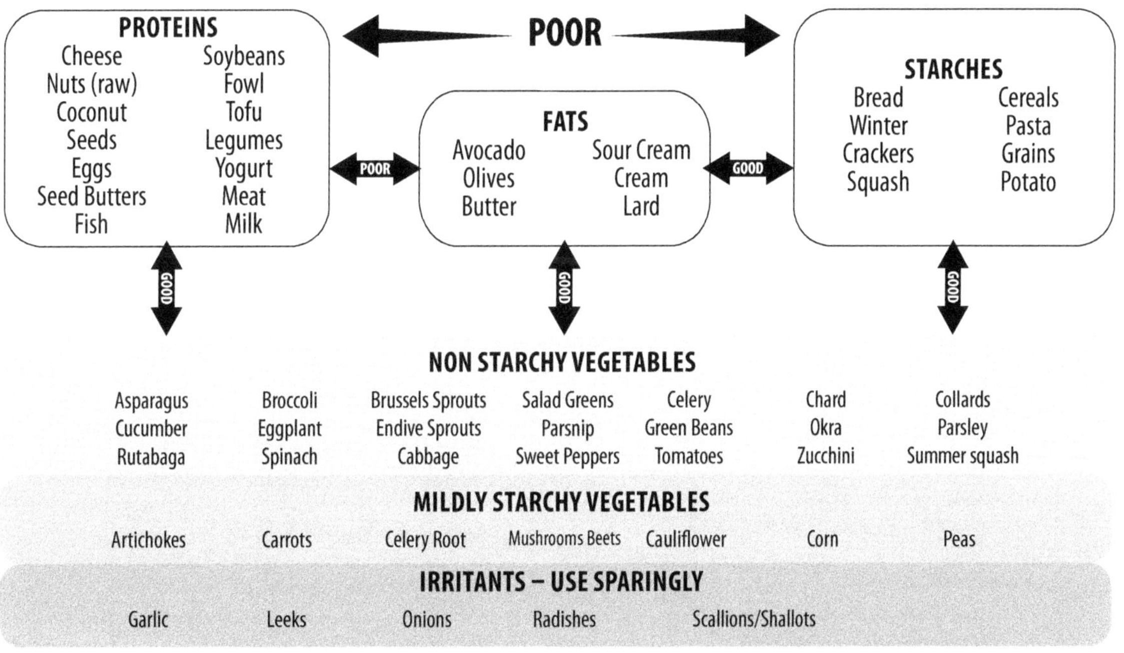

Eat fruit by itself on an empty stomach. Let 20-30 minutes elapse after eating fruit before eating other foods. Wait another 3 hours after eating cooked food before eating fruit again.

ACID FRUIT
Blackberries, Plums (sour), Pineapple, Pomegranate, Citrus (lemon, lime, orange, grapefruit, etc)

SUB-ACID FRUIT
Apple, Kiwi, Apricot, Nectarine, Blueberries, Papaya, Cherries, Peach, Fresh figs, Pear, Grapes, Plums (sweet)

SWEET FRUIT
Bananas, Dates, Dried Fruit, Raisins, Persimmon
(Ideally sweet fruit should be eaten after other fruits)

MELONS
Ideally melon of any kind should be eaten alone or before other fruits

Endnotes

1. Tolle, Eckhart (1999). The Power of Now: A Guide to Spiritual Enlightenment. P.O. Box 62084, Vancouver, B.C., Canada, V6I 4A3 : Namaste Publishing.
2. Trudeau, Kevin, (2009). Your Wish is Your Command, Global Information Network, Hinsdale, IL
3. (Lee .S Gross, Earl S Ford, and Simin Lui, (2004) The American Journal of Clinical Nutrition).
4. Phillips, Bill (1999). Body For Life. New York, NY, Harper Collins Publishers.
5. King, J. Brad. The Fat Wars Un-Diet Plan: Seven Steps to Awaken Your Body. Hillsburg, ON, Health Venture Publications
6. Kapit, Macey, Meisami (2000). The Physiology Coloring Book. USA, Addison Wesley Longman, Inc.
7. Richards, Dr. James B.(2010). Wired or Success, Programmed for Failure. Newburg, PA: Mile Stones International Publishers.
8. Chris Kresser, (2013), Gut Health.
9. http://www.peterson-handwriting.com/Publications/PDF_versions/ReviewSections123.pdf
10. Trudeau, Kevin, (2009). Your Wish is Your Command, Global Information Network, Hinsdale, IL
11. Eker, T. Harv, (2005). Secrets of the Millionaire Mind, Harper Collins Publishers, New York, NY,
12. Grout, Pam, (2013). E2, Hay House Inc., USA
13. http://www.fredalanwolf.com
14. Ziglar, Zig, (1975). See You At The Top, Pelican Publishing Company Inc., Gretna, Louisiana
15. Trudeau, Kevin, (2009). Your Wish is Your Command, Global Information Network, Hinsdale, IL
16. Eker, T.Harv, (2005). Secrets of the Millionaire Mind, (pp.58-59).Harper Collins Publishers, New York, NY,
17. http://gochemless.com/top-10-dangers-of-swimming-pool-chlorine/
18. Grout, Pam, (2013). E2, Hay House Inc., USA
19. Trudeau, Kevin, (2009). Masters Teaching Level One, Global Information Network, Hinsdale, IL
20. Ziglar, Zig, (1975). See You At The Top, Pelican Publishing Company Inc., Gretna, Louisiana
21. xii http://lowcarbdiets.about.com/library/blbodyfatcharts.htm
22. xiii http://www.hsph.harvard.edu/nutritionsource/alcohol-full-story/#what_is_moderate
23. King, J. Brad. The Fat Wars Un-Diet Plan: Seven Steps to Awaken Your Body. (pp. 34-35) Hillsburg, ON, Health Venture Publications.
24. http://www.bodybuilding.com/fun/fat_loss_training_wars.htm
25. http://www.bodybuilding.com/fun/fat_loss_training_wars.htm
26. http://www.volac.com/lifestyle-ingredients/why-whey/market-sectors/whey-protein-and-muscle-synthesis
27. http://www.volac.com/lifestyle-ingredients/why-whey/market-sectors/whey-protein-and-muscle-synthesis
28. Tolle, Eckhart (1999).. The Power of Now: A Guide to Spiritual Enlightenment. P.O. Box 62084, Vancouver, B.C., Canada, V6I 4A3: Namaste Publishing.
29. Spalding, Baird T. (1948). Life and Teaching of the Masters of the Far East, Volume 4, (pp. 172-173). Camarillo, CA: DeVross & Company, Publisher
30. Spalding, Baird T. (1948). Life and Teaching of the Masters of the Far East, Volume 4, Camarillo, CA: DeVross & Company, Publisher
31. Vincent Peale, Norman (1952). The Power of Positive Thinking. New York, Fawcett Columbine Book and Ballantine Books Publishing.
32. Watson, Brenda, N.D. and Leonard Smith, M.D.(2003). Gut Solutions: Natural Solutions to Your Digestive Problems. Clearwater, FL..: Renew Life Press and Information Services
33. Anderson, Richard, N.D., N.M.D., (1988). Cleanse & Purify Thyself, Medford, OR, Christobe Publishing, pg.

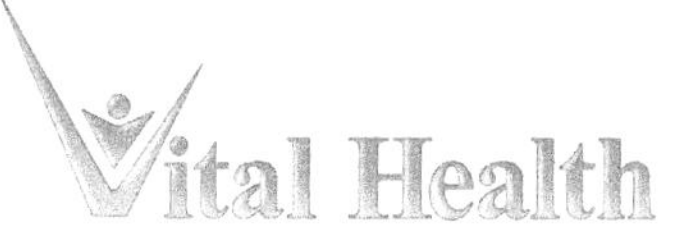

34. Turner, Natasha. (2010). The Hormone Diet: Lose Fat.Gain Strength. Live Younger Longer. Toronto, Canada: Random House of Canada Limited.
35. http://www.paleoforwomen.com/the-estrogen-dominance-post-where-its-coming-from-and-what-to-do-about-it/
36. Turner, Natasha. (2010). The Hormone Diet: Lose Fat.Gain Strength. Live Younger Longer. Toronto, Canada: Random House of Canada Limited.
37. Mitrea, Liliana Stadler (2005). Pathology and Nutrition: A Guide for Professionals. Canada: CSNN Publishing, A Division of Canadian School of Natural Nutrition Inc.
38. Jensen, Bernard, D.C.(1981). Tissue Cleansing Through Bowel Management.Escondido, CA, Bernard Jensen Enterprises
39. http://www.webnat.com/articles/MucusAbout.asp
40. http://draxe.com/canola-oil-gm/
41. Turner, Natasha. (2010). The Hormone Diet: Lose Fat.Gain Strength. Live Younger Longer. Toronto, Canada: Random House of Canada Limited.
42. Harvey and Marilyn Diamond, (1985), Fit For Life, pp 63.
43. http://articles.mercola.com/sites/articles/archive/2010/10/13/soy-controversy-and-health-effects.aspx
44. Kyssa, Natasha (2009).The Simply Raw: Living Foods, Detox Manual.Vancouver, B.C.
45. Fuhrman, Joel, M.D. (2012), Eat For Health. Flemington, N.J.: Gift of Health Press.
46. http://drhedberg.com/blog/wp-content/uploads/2010/06/7-Steps-to-Optimal-Health.pdf
47. http://www.medicalnewstoday.com/articles/266069.php
48. Diamond, Harvey & Marilyn, (1985). Fit For Life (pp.27). New York: N.Y.
49. http://www.precisionnutrition.com/digesting-whole-vs-processed-foods
50. Ali, Elvis, N.D., Floener, Pam, P.T., R.M.A., Garshowitz, David, Bsc.,Phm., Grant, George, M.Sc., M.Ed., Ed.D., Ko, Gordon, M.D., Levy, Joseph, Ph.D., Marshall, Dorothy, Ph.D., Pettle, Alvin., M.D.(2000). The All In One Guide to Natural Remedies and Supplements. Ages Publications, Niagara Falls, New York.
51. Kean, Maureen & Calbom, Cherie (1992). Juicing For Life: A Guide to the Health Benefits of Fresh Fruit and Vegetable Juicing. U.S.A.: Avery a member of Penguin Putnam Inc.
52. http://botanical.com/
53. http://parasitecleanse.com/parasites.htm
54. http://www.huldaclarkzappers.com/php2/parasitecleanse.php
55. http://www.frequencyrising.com/parasitecleanse.htm
56. http://emedicine.medscape.com/article/815051-overview#a0101
57. www.epa.gov/oppt/existingchemicals/pubs/actionplans/pfcs.html
58. http://www.advancedbionutritionals.com/Products/PectaSol-Detox-Formula.html
59. http://www.thefreedictionary.com/PCB
60. http://www.justcleansing.com/heavy-metal-cleanse.htm
61. http://www.blenderbabes.com/blender-babes-101/blender-babes-how-to-tips/how-to-wash-fruits-vegetables-and-remove-pesticides-with-diy-homemade-recipes/
62. http://www.newhealthguide.org/Sesame-Oil-Benefits.html
63. Turner, Natasha. (2010). The Hormone Diet: Lose Fat.Gain Strength. Live Younger Longer. Toronto, Canada: Random House of Canada Limited
64. http://www.studio-figura.co.uk/en/five-golden-rules-of-drinking-water
65. Harvey and Marilyn Diamond, (1985), Fit For Life, pp 44-45
66. Natasha Kyssa, (2009), The Simply Raw Living Foods Detox Manual, pp. 52-53
67. Lagerquist, Ron & Coghill, Thomas (1996). God's Banquet Table. Pp.49-50
68. Harvey and Marilyn Diamond, (1985), Fit For Life, pp. 40-42
69. http://articles.mercola.com/sites/articles/archive/2011/05/02/is-sugar-toxic.aspx
70. Harvey and Marilyn Diamond, (1985), Fit For Life, pp 65-66
71. http://health.howstuffworks.com/wellness/food-nutrition/vitamin-supplements/body-absorb-vitamins.htm
72. Harvey and Marilyn Diamond, (1985), Fit For Life, pp 65-66
73. http://www.ion.ac.uk/information/onarchives/food.com, Dr. Hay, ION Archives (Spring 1994)
74. Lagerquist, Ronald & Coghill, Thomas (1996) God's Banquet Table, pp. 169-175
75. http://www.livescience.com/39353-eggs-dont-deserve-bad-reputation.html
76. Pauline, B. Gunther, The Divine Prescription and Science of Health and Healing, p.212
77. B. Esmarck, J. L., Andersen*, S. Olsen, E. A. Richter†, M. Mizuno‡ and M Kjær, Timing of post exercise protein intake is important for muscle hypertrophy with resistance training in elderly humans
78. Harvey and Marilyn Diamond, (1985), Fit For Life, pp 52-53
79. Paul Vessel and Alexandra Devarenne, University of California Cooperative Extension
80. http://thechronicleflask.wordpress.com/2013/08/28/amazing-alkaline-lemons
81. http://drleonardcoldwell.com/2013/03/13/aged-balsamic-vinegar-health-benefit
82. http://www.nutrition-and-you.com/parsley.html
83. http://juicing-for-health.com/basic-nutrition/healing-vegetables/health-benefits-of-cilantro.html
84. Klaunig E., James, Kamendulis, Lisa M., Hocevar, Barbara A., Oxidative Stress and Oxidative Damage in Carcinogenesis, Toxicologic Pathology, Sage Journal
85. http://healthyeating.sfgate.com/benefits-hummus-4608.html
86. http://healthyeating.sfgate.com/body-excess-vitamin-b-c-might-consume-3056.html
87. Grant, Dr. George (2000), The All in One Guide to Natural Remedies and Supplements, (p. 70), Adi, Gaia, Esalen Publication Inc.

88. Sullivan, Karen (1998), Vitamins and Minerals, and Illustrated Guide, Element Books Limited, pp. 31-37
89. Grant, Dr. George (2000), The All in One Guide to Natural Remedies and Supplements,(p.70), Adi, Gaia, Esalen Publication Inc.
90. Sullivan, Karen (1998), Vitamins and Minerals, and Illustrated Guide, Element Books Limited, pp. 38-39
91. http://sodiumbreakup.heart.org/sodium-411/sea-salt-vs-table-salt/, American Heart Association
92. http://umm.edu/health/medical/altmed/supplement/omega3-fatty-acids,
93. University of Maryland Medical Center
94. Kapit, Macey, Meisami (2000). The Physiology Coloring Book. San Francisco, CA.: Benjamin/Cummings Science Publishing. (p.130)
95. Graham, Paul (2011). Nutrition & Lifestyle Coach Course Manual. (p.19) Ottawa, ON: Peak Performance.
96. http://lowcarbdiets.about.com/od/nutrition/a/starch.htm
97. Lagerquist, Ron & Coghill, Thomas (1996) God's Banquet Table, (pp. 250-251)
98. http://www.fitday.com/fitness-articles/nutrition/healthy-eating/the-nutrition-of-whole-wheat-pasta.html#b
99. Lagerquist, Ron & Coghill, Thomas (1996) God's Banquet Table, pp.111-112
100. http://www.nutritionexpress.com/article+index/authors/mark+g+taylor+ms/showarticle.aspx?articleid=896
101. William, G. Helferich, the Journal of Nutrition, November 2001, National Institute of Health, University of Illinois
102. http://growingnaturals.com/knowledge/our-proteins/why-rice-protein/
103. https://www.baselinenutritionals.com/products/nutribody-protein.php
104. http://ndosupps.com/anti-aging-muscles/
105. Oster, K., Oster, J., and Ross, D. Immune Response to Bovine Xanthine Oxidase in Atherosclerotic Patients. American Laboratory, August, 1974, 41-47
106. http://dancingdogfarm.com/category/living-food/
107. http://ybertaud9.wordpress.com/2013/02/20/butternut-squash-soup-health-benefits/
108. http://www.amazon.com/Pacific-Natural-Foods-Organic-16-Ounce/dp/B000LKU1TO
109. Lagerquist, Ron & Coghill, Thomas(1996) God's Banquet Table, pp. 121-122
110. Biochemical and Biophysical Research Communication, 2005
111. http://www.naturalfoodbenefits.com/display.asp?CAT=3&ID=89
112. http://www.mercola.com/beef/health_benefits.htm
113. http://www.oneresult.com/articles/nutrition/nutritional-benefits-wild-fish
114. http://www.montanaelk.com/nutrition.html
115. http://ods.od.nih.gov/factsheets/Folate-HealthProfessional/#h10
116. http://www.mindbodygreen.com/0-4408/Top-10-Health-Benefits-of-Eating-Kale.html, Alison Lewis, April 2, 2012
117. Lagerquist, Ron & Coghill, Thomas(1996) God's Banquet Table, pp. 102-103
118. http://www.bodybuilding.com/fun/glutamine.htm
119. http://www.bodybuilding.com/fun/bcaas-the-many-benefits-of-amino-acids.html
120. http://www.muscleandfitness.com/supplements/build-muscle/everything-you-ever-wanted-know-about-creatine
121. http://www.themacateam.com/maca-benefits
122. http://www.bengreenfieldfitness.com/2013/07/how-much-carbohydrate-protein-and-fat-you-need/
123. http://www.sharecare.com/health/minerals-nutrition-diet/
124. http://www.medicinenet.com/diabetic_diet/page8.htm#meat_and_meat_substitutes
125. http://diabetes.about.com/od/diabeticmealplansmenus/a/Low-Fat_1400-Calorie-Meal_Plan.htm
126. Beliveau, Richard, Ph.D., Gingras, Denis, Ph.D.(2006). Cooking with Foods that fight Cancer. Toronto, Canada, McClelland & Stewart Ltd.
127. Beliveau, Richard, Ph.D., Gingras, Denis, Ph.D.(2006). Cooking with Foods that fight Cancer.
128. (p. 110). Toronto, Canada, McClelland & Stewart Ltd.
129. Beliveau, Richard, Ph.D., Gingras, Denis, Ph.D.(2006). Cooking with Foods that fight Cancer.
130. (pp.112-113). Toronto, Canada, McClelland & Stewart Ltd.
131. Beliveau, Richard, Ph.D., Gingras, Denis, Ph.D.(2006). Cooking with Foods that fight Cancer.
132. (pp. 61-65). Toronto, Canada, McClelland & Stewart Ltd.
133. Beliveau, Richard, Ph.D., Gingras, Denis, Ph.D.(2006). Cooking with Foods that fight Cancer.
134. (pp.69-73). Toronto, Canada, McClelland & Stewart Ltd.
135. Beliveau, Richard, Ph.D., Gingras, Denis, Ph.D.(2006). Cooking with Foods that fight Cancer.
136. (p. 115). Toronto, Canada, McClelland & Stewart Ltd.
137. Beliveau, Richard, Ph.D., Gingras, Denis, Ph.D.(2006). Cooking with Foods that fight Cancer. (p. 116-117). Toronto, Canada, McClelland & Stewart Ltd.
138. Beliveau, Richard, Ph.D., Gingras, Denis, Ph.D.(2006). Cooking with Foods that fight Cancer.
139. (pp.86-91)Toronto, Canada, McClelland & Stewart Ltd.
140. Beliveau, Richard, Ph.D., Gingras, Denis, Ph.D.(2006). Cooking with Foods that fight Cancer.
141. (pp. 93-101). Toronto, Canada, McClelland & Stewart Ltd.
142. Beliveau, Richard, Ph.D., Gingras, Denis, Ph.D.(2006). Cooking with Foods that fight Cancer. (pp.102-103). Toronto, Canada, McClelland & Stewart Ltd.
143. Beliveau, Richard, Ph.D., Gingras, Denis, Ph.D.(2006). Cooking with Foods that fight Cancer. (pp. 104-105). Toronto, Canada, McClelland & Stewart Ltd.
144. Beliveau, Richard, Ph.D., Gingras, Denis, Ph.D.(2006). Cooking with Foods that fight Cancer.
145. (pp. 108-109)Toronto, Canada, McClelland & Stewart Ltd.

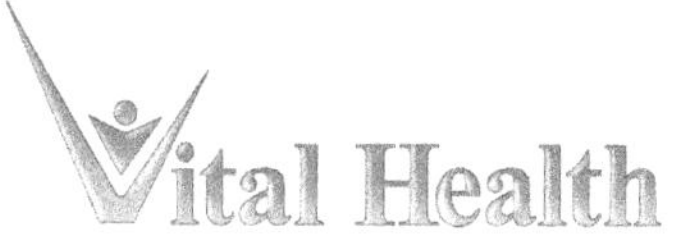

146. Beliveau, Richard, Ph.D., Gingras, Denis, Ph.D.(2006). Cooking with Foods that fight Cancer.
147. (pp. 80-83). Toronto, Canada, McClelland & Stewart Ltd.
148. Page, Linda, N.D., Ph.D. April 2002 Natural Solutions for Hypothyroidism. The Messenger.
149. http://www.diethealthclub.com/health-issues-and-diet/hyperthyroidism.html
150. Tanguay, Linda Ann Frances, Certified Bio-Feedback Consultant (2011). Hypothyroidism Chart. Ottawa, ON. http://www.lowthyroidhelp.com/foods-that-help-the-thyroid-gland.html; http://al-health-care.com/thyroid-foods-print.htm; http://www.buzzle.com/articles/hypothyroidism-natural-treatment.html; http://www.buzzle.com/articles/iodine-rich-foods.html;
151. http://www.iodine4health.com/research/iodine_in_food_table.htm; http://www.mayoclinic.com/health/hypothyroidism/DS00353/DSECTION=symptoms; http://www.squidoo.com/hashimotos_thyroiditis; http://health4bodymindandsoul.com/2011/02/problem-with-thyroid-and-home-remedies-treatment
152. http://www.womens-health-advice.com/yeast-infections/candida-diet-plan.html#Diet
153. https://crohnspainfreefoods.com/?utm_source=bing&utm_medium=cpc&utm_term=+diet%20for%20+crohn%27s%20+disease&utm_content=e&utm_campaign=Crohns-%2BSearch%2BOpt%2BADW
154. http://www.healthline.com/health-slideshow/crohns-disease-power-foods#1
155. http://www.webmd.com/digestive-disorders/diverticular-disease?page=2
156. http://www.naturalnews.com/037995_diet_diverticulitis_dietary_fiber.html
157. http://www.nhs.uk/Conditions/Diverticular-disease-and-diverticulitis/Pages/Prevention.aspx
158. https://sites.google.com/site/diverticulardiseasesymposium/low-residue-diet
159. http://www.nlm.nih.gov/medlineplus/ency/patientinstructions/000200.htm
160. Watson, Brenda, N.D. and Leonard Smith, M.D.(2003). Gut Solutions: Natural Solutions to Your Digestive Problems. Clearwater, FL..: Renew Life Press and Information Services
161. http://www.webmd.com/ibs/features/finding-right-diet-ibs
162. http://www.webmd.com/ibs/features/finding-right-diet-ibs
163. Watson, Brenda, N.D. and Leonard Smith, M.D.(2003). Gut Solutions: Natural Solutions to Your Digestive Problems. Clearwater, FL..: Renew Life Press and Information Services
164. http://articles.mercola.com/sites/articles/archive/2014/04/28/acid-reflux-ulcer-treatment.aspx
165. http://jcp.bmj.com/content/45/2/135.abstract
166. Watson, Brenda, N.D. and Leonard Smith, M.D.(2003). Gut Solutions: Natural Solutions to Your Digestive Problems. Clearwater, FL..: Renew Life Press and Information Services
167. Jonathan V. wright, MD and Lane Lenard, PHD, Why Stomach Acid is Good for You, M. Evans and Company, Inc., 2001, P.92
168. Ibid.,p. 48.
169. Dr. John Mckenna, Hard to Stomach, Newleaf, 2002, p. 121
170. Ibid.
171. http://www.sustainablebabysteps.com/natural-antifungal.html
172. http://www.medicalnewstoday.com/articles/266016.php
173. http://www.livestrong.com/article/110565-dgl-licorice-acid-reflux/
174. http://www.aloelife.com/aloe-education/health-benefits-of-aloevera/
175. Watson, Brenda, N.D. and Leonard Smith, M.D.(2003). Gut Solutions: Natural Solutions to Your Digestive Problems. Clearwater, FL..: Renew Life Press and Information Services, p. 212
176. http://skipthepie.org/vegetables-and-vegetable-products/potatoes-russet-flesh-and-skin-raw/
177. Wiatt, Carrie.(2008) Nutrition Plan Eating For Power Performance.Beverly Hills, CA: Product Partners, LLC.
178. Tahiliani, Marc, N.D.(2012). PureTrim Mediterranean Wellness System. AwarenessLife WorldWide
179. Wiatt, Carrie.(2008) Nutrition Plan Eating For Power Performance.Beverly Hills, CA: Product Partners, LLC.
180. http://www.ewg.org/research/healthy-home-tips/tip-6-skip-non-stick-avoid-dangers-teflon
181. http://www.vitamindcouncil.org/about-vitamin-d/how-do-i-get-the-vitamin-d-my-body-needs/
182. http://www.nationalnutrition.ca/detail.aspx?ID=260
183. http://www.merckmanuals.com/professional/nutritional_disorders/vitamin_deficiency_dependency_and_toxicity/vitamin_a.html?qt=nutritional%20disorders&alt=sh
184. http://www.webmd.com/vitamins-and-supplements/lifestyle-guide-11/supplement-guide-chromium
185. http://www.naturalfactors.com/caen/products/detail/2876/multi-enzyme
186. http://www.peertrainer.com/health/CoQ10_what_you_need_to_know.aspx
187. http://www.chm.bris.ac.uk/motm/chlorophyll/chlorophyll_h.htm
188. http://www.genuinehealth.com/store/greens#.VK84tivF-So
189. http://www.drugs.com/npp/echinacea.html
190. https://beesweetontario.com/pages/Creams.html
191. http://www.phytochemicals.info/phytochemicals/isothiocyanates.php
192. http://authoritynutrition.com/top-10-evidence-based-health-benefits-of-green-tea/
193. http://www.cnn.com/2013/02/26/health/five-things-olive-oil/
194. http://www.medicalnewstoday.com/articles/270406.php
195. Turner, Natasha. (2010). The Hormone Diet: Lose Fat.Gain Strength. Live Younger Longer. Toronto, Canada: Random House of Canada Limited.
196. http://www.care2.com/greenliving/8-health-benefits-of-almonds-king-of-n
197. Turner, Natasha. (2010). The Hormone Diet: Lose Fat, Gain Strength, Live Younger Longer. Toronto, Canada: Random House of Canada Limited.

CPSIA information can be obtained
at www.ICGtesting.com
Printed in the USA
BVHW011104231221
623841BV00013B/200